AF614688

New Perspectives on Asthma

Edited by Xiaoyan Dong and Nanbert Zhong

Published in London, United Kingdom

New Perspectives on Asthma
http://dx.doi.org/10.5772/intechopen.101004
Edited by Xiaoyan Dong and Nanbert Zhong

Contributors
Maha Dardouri, Manel Mallouli, Jihene Bouguila, Jihene Sahli, Chekib Zedini, Ali Mtiraoui, Christian Castillo Latorre, Alba D. Rivera Diaz, Sulimar Morales Colon, Vanessa Fonseca Ferrer, Onix Cantres Fonseca, William Rodriguez Cintron, Luis Gerena Montano, Ilean Lamboy Hernandez, Mariana Mercader Perez, Chen Hao, Cui Yubao, Zhu Rongfei, Feidie Li, Xiaoyan Dong, Chao Wang, Ran Zhao, Yanhua Niu

© The Editor(s) and the Author(s) 2023

The rights of the editor(s) and the author(s) have been asserted in accordance with the Copyright, Designs and Patents Act 1988. All rights to the book as a whole are reserved by INTECHOPEN LIMITED. The book as a whole (compilation) cannot be reproduced, distributed or used for commercial or non-commercial purposes without INTECHOPEN LIMITED's written permission. Enquiries concerning the use of the book should be directed to INTECHOPEN LIMITED rights and permissions department (permissions@intechopen.com).

Violations are liable to prosecution under the governing Copyright Law.

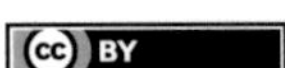

Individual chapters of this publication are distributed under the terms of the Creative Commons Attribution 3.0 Unported License which permits commercial use, distribution and reproduction of the individual chapters, provided the original author(s) and source publication are appropriately acknowledged. If so indicated, certain images may not be included under the Creative Commons license. In such cases users will need to obtain permission from the license holder to reproduce the material. More details and guidelines concerning content reuse and adaptation can be found at http://www.intechopen.com/copyright-policy.html.

Notice

Statements and opinions expressed in the chapters are these of the individual contributors and not necessarily those of the editors or publisher. No responsibility is accepted for the accuracy of information contained in the published chapters. The publisher assumes no responsibility for any damage or injury to persons or property arising out of the use of any materials, instructions, methods or ideas contained in the book.

First published in London, United Kingdom, 2023 by IntechOpen
IntechOpen is the global imprint of INTECHOPEN LIMITED, registered in England and Wales, registration number: 11086078, 5 Princes Gate Court, London, SW7 2QJ, United Kingdom

British Library Cataloguing-in-Publication Data
A catalogue record for this book is available from the British Library

Additional hard and PDF copies can be obtained from orders@intechopen.com

New Perspectives on Asthma
Edited by Xiaoyan Dong and Nanbert Zhong
p. cm.
Print ISBN 978-1-80356-302-2
Online ISBN 978-1-80356-303-9
eBook (PDF) ISBN 978-1-80356-304-6

We are IntechOpen, the world's leading publisher of Open Access books

Built by scientists, for scientists

6,600+
Open access books available

178,000+
International authors and editors

195M+
Downloads

156
Countries delivered to

Our authors are among the
Top 1%
most cited scientists

12.2%
Contributors from top 500 universities

WEB OF SCIENCE™

Selection of our books indexed in the Book Citation Index in Web of Science™ Core Collection (BKCI)

Interested in publishing with us?
Contact book.department@intechopen.com

Numbers displayed above are based on latest data collected.
For more information visit www.intechopen.com

For EU product safety concerns:
IN TECH d.o.o., Prolaz Marije Krucifikse Kozulić 3, 51000 Rijeka, Croatia,
info@intechopen.com or visit our website at intechopen.com.

Meet the editors

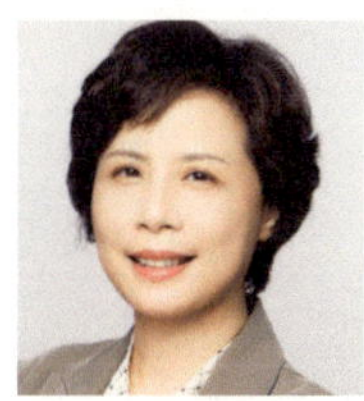

Xiaoyan Dong, MD, is an esteemed master's supervisor and serves as the director of the Department of Respiratory Medicine, Shanghai Children's Hospital, China. She obtained her MD from the School of Medicine, Shanghai Jiaotong University, China, and has pursued additional training at renowned institutions such as Yale University School of Medicine, USA, and the New York State Institute of Developmental Disabilities. Dr. Dong holds leadership roles and membership in various national pediatric associations, including the Chinese Medical Association and the Chinese Maternal and Child Health Association. With a specialization in the prevention and treatment of pediatric respiratory diseases, Dr. Dong has made significant contributions to her field. Her expertise is reflected in the publication of more than sixty academic papers and books. She has also played a pivotal role in leading and participating in numerous national and municipal research projects related to pediatric respiratory diseases. Dr. Dong's dedication to advancing medical knowledge and improving patient care has earned her recognition and respect within the medical community.

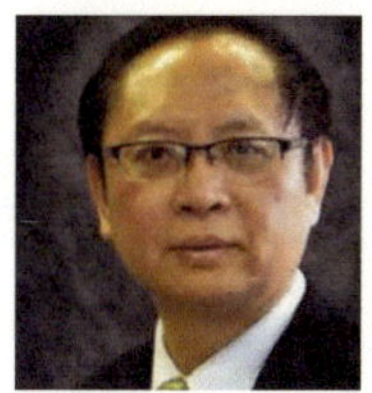

Dr. Nanber Zhong is the founder and director of the Peking University Center of Medical Genetics, China, as well as the founder professor and chairman of the Department of Medical Genetics, Peking University Health Science Center, China. Dr. Zhong's research focuses on investigating the pathogenic impact of gene–environment interactions during intrauterine development on pregnancy outcomes and fetal–child development. He has an impressive publication record with more than 170 research articles published in peer-reviewed journals, including Lancet and Nature Genetics. Notably, his research studies have received funding from reputable institutions such as the National Institutes of Health (NIH), the March of Dimes Foundation, the Batten Disease Support and Research Association, and the New York State Research Foundation for Mental Hygiene.

Contents

Preface

Bronchial asthma is a chronic respiratory disease that poses a significant threat to the physical and mental well-being of children, placing a heavy burden on both families and society. The global prevalence of asthma is on the rise, making it crucial for pediatric healthcare professionals to prioritize the prevention and treatment of this condition. In recent years, experts in pediatric medicine have dedicated extensive research to understanding the causes, pathogenesis, clinical prevention, treatment, health education, and awareness of asthma. The objective is to ensure that healthcare personnel, children, and their families have accurate knowledge and can effectively prevent asthma.

While this research has yielded positive results, challenges persist due to the unequal distribution of medical resources, varying levels of disease prevention and treatment, and disparities in social development and disease knowledge. Consequently, healthcare professionals often lack comprehensive knowledge about asthma and require ongoing education regarding its diagnosis, treatment, and underlying mechanisms. Thus, there is an urgent need to enhance and broaden the understanding of asthmatic disease.

This book summarizes recent perspectives on the pathogenesis of asthma, advancements in its diagnosis and treatment, epigenetic and biomarker studies pertaining to asthma, the correlation between environmental factors, occupational hazards, and asthma development, as well as family education and asthma management. We firmly believe that this book will contribute to the promotion of asthma prevention, treatment, and research into its underlying mechanisms. Our sincere wish is for children with asthma worldwide to achieve a better quality of life.

Xiaoyan Dong, M.D., Ph.D.
Chair,
Department of Respiratory Medicine,
Shanghai Children's Hospital,
Shanghai Jiao Tong University School of Medicine,
Shanghai, China

Dr. Nanbert Zhong
New York State Institute for Basic Research in Developmental Disabilities,
New York, United States of America

Chapter 1

Introductory Chapter: New Understandings of Asthma

Ran Zhao and Xiaoyan Dong

1. Introduction

Asthma is a heterogeneous disease characterized by chronic airway inflammation and airway hyperresponsiveness, and the main lesion site is bronchi. It is a threat to public health worldwide and affects people of all ages. According to relevant data, it is conservatively estimated that there are at least 300 million asthma patients in the world, and 380,000 people die of asthma every year. Asthma has become a serious public health problem, bringing great pressure to individuals, families and the society. At the same time, the incidence of asthma is also one of the fastest rising diseases in the world. Data show that the overall prevalence of asthma in both adults and children has been increasing worldwide for the past 20 years. At present, the prevalence of asthma varies greatly among countries in the world, ranging from 0.3–17%, and the incidence of asthma varies in different regions and genders within the same country. Generally speaking, the incidence of asthma is higher in developed countries than in developing countries and higher in urban areas than in rural areas [1, 2].

The mechanism of asthma is complicated, and its pathogenesis has not been fully understood. Currently, asthma is considered to be a heterogeneous disease with the combined effects of gene and environment [3]. Asthma is a polygenic disease, and hundreds of asthma susceptibility gene loci have been found, which are related to the molecular mechanism and pathophysiological manifestations. Epigenetics regulate asthma between environmental and genetic factors through DNA methylation, histone modification, and regulation of non-coding RNA [4]. At the same time, the complex role of airway and gut microbiome in the development and severity of asthma has also been recognized [3].

2. New understandings of asthma in definitions, phenotypes and treatments

In recent years, thanks to the continuous explorations and understandings of the pathogenesis of asthma, as well as high-quality clinical trials and real-world data, the recommended treatment strategies of various countries are updated frequently, and new drugs for asthma treatment keep emerging. The field of asthma treatment develops rapidly.

First, the definition of asthma is constantly being updated. The 2021 update of GINA no longer distinguishes between intermittent and mild persistent asthma and refers to both as mild asthma. The preferred treatment for mild asthma is updated to low-dose ICS/formoterol on demand [5]. However, the Spanish Asthma Management

Guidelines (GEMA) [6], published in 2021, differ from GINA in their definition and treatment guidelines for mild asthma, which retain intermittent asthma and can be treated with one of three options: SABA, or low dose ICS/formoterol, or low dose ICS/salbutamol, and GEMA continues to recommend daily maintenance of low dose ICS as the preferred treatment for mild persistent asthma. The definition and treatment strategies for mild asthma are still controversial, and more evidence and research is needed to gain more agreement. Therefore, GINA 2022 recommends that the term 'mild asthma' should generally be avoided in clinical practice, but if it was used, patients should be alerted to the risk of acute attacks of severe asthma and the need for ICS-containing treatment.

Second, with the deepening understanding of the mechanism of asthma, the phenotypes of asthma are also changing. More and more clinicians believe that asthma cannot be simply divided into allergic type and non-allergic type. In many asthmatic patients, chronic airway inflammation is driven by Th2 or ILC2 cells that produce IL-4, IL-5, and IL-13, and these type 2 cytokines and promote typical features of the disease, such as eosinophilia accumulation, hypersecretion of mucus, bronchial hyperresponsiveness, increased IgE production and susceptibility to exacerbation. However, only half of asthmatics have this type 2 high feature, whereas type 2 low asthma is more associated with obesity, high neutrophils and a lack of response to corticosteroids, the main drug used to treat asthma [7]. So that, in recent years, the phenotype of asthma has evolved into endotype: type 2 high (essentially eosinophilic type) and type 2 low (non-eosinophilic, sometimes neutrophilic, and metabolic). The therapeutic targets of different endogenous inflammatory pathways have become the new focus of drug research and development for asthma.

Finally, asthma treatments are constantly being updated. Among them, the emergence of new targets in both type 2 high and type 2 low inflammatory pathways has led to more strategies for treatment. In the year of 2022, GINA added TSLP target antibody into the treatment program. Up to now, there have been four types of target drugs approved internationally. Three biological antibodies have been produced to target IL-5, Mepolizumab, an IgG1 antibody directed against IL-5 [8], cells expressing the IL-5 receptor alpha chain such as eosinophils and basophils [9, 10]. The target of IL-4RA inhibition is Dupilumab, which was first used in eosinophilic asthma and is also effective in non-eosinophilic asthma patients [11]. Currently, IL-9 inhibitors have not been shown to be effective in patients with moderate to severe asthma [12]. Omalizumab, a biologic agent targeting IgE, has been widely used in the clinic, but only about 70% of children and adults treated with Omalizumab showed a good response to treatment [13]. Epithelium-derived inflammatory cytokines include IL-1, IL-33, IL-25 and TSLP, among which biologics targeting IL-33 and TSLP are more advanced, and results of the clinical trials have only been published for TSLP. Tezepelumab (AMG 157/MEDI9929) is a humanized monoclonal antibody to TSLP that can be applied to both type 2 high and type 2 low severe asthma [14]. At present, in addition to the development of new drugs and clinical trials, several issues still need to be addressed in biotarget therapy, including the length of time that severe patients need to be treated with biologic agents; the risk assessment of immunogenicity of monoclonal antibodies, and more data are needed in special populations.

3. Summary

With the continuous exploration of the pathogenesis of asthma and the development and analysis of various clinical trials, the diagnosis and treatment of asthma, as well as the development of drugs, are constantly updated and improved. This book summarized recent researches on the diagnosis and treatment of asthma and its mechanisms. In the future, with more comprehensive and in-depth explorations of inflammatory pathways in asthma and evidence-based supports from high-quality clinical studies, the treatment of asthma will continue to make great strides forward for the benefit of asthma patients.

Author details

Ran Zhao and Xiaoyan Dong*
Department of Respiratory Medicine, Shanghai Children's Hospital, Shanghai Jiao Tong University School of Medicine, Shanghai, China

*Address all correspondence to: dongxy@shchildren.com.cn

IntechOpen

© 2023 The Author(s). Licensee IntechOpen. This chapter is distributed under the terms of the Creative Commons Attribution License (http://creativecommons.org/licenses/by/3.0), which permits unrestricted use, distribution, and reproduction in any medium, provided the original work is properly cited. (cc) BY

References

[1] Global initiative for asthma. Global Strategy for Asthma Management and Prevention. 2022

[2] Holgate ST, Wenzel S, Postma DS, Weiss ST, Renz H, Sly PD. Asthma. Nature Reviews. Disease Primers. 2015;**1**(1):15025. DOI: 10.1038/nrdp.2015.25

[3] Ntontsi P, Photiades A, Zervas E, Xanthou G, Samitas K. Genetics and epigenetics in asthma. International Journal of Molecular Sciences. 2021;**22**(5):2412. DOI: 10.3390/ijms22052412

[4] Cevhertas L, Ogulur I, Maurer DJ, Burla D, Ding M, Jansen K, et al. Advances and recent developments in asthma in 2020. Allergy. 2020;**75**(12):3124-3146. DOI: 10.1111/all.14607 Epub 2020 Oct 16

[5] Global initiative for asthma. Global Strategy for Asthma Management and Prevention. 2021

[6] Plaza V, Blanco M, García G, et al. Highlights of the Spanish Asthma Guidelines (GEMA), version 5.0. Novedades y otros aspectos destacados de la Guía Española para el Manejo del Asma (GEMA), versión 5.0. Arch Bronconeumol (Engl Ed). 2021;**57**(1):11-12. DOI: 10.1016/j.arbres.2020.10.003

[7] Hammad H, Lambrecht BN. The basic immunology of asthma. Cell. 2021;**184**(6):1469-1485. DOI: 10.1016/j.cell.2021.02.016 Epub 2021 Mar 11. Erratum in: Cell. 2021 Apr 29;184(9):2521-2522

[8] Leckie MJ, ten Brinke A, Khan J, Diamant Z, O'Connor BJ, Walls CM, et al. Effects of an interleukin-5 blocking monoclonal antibody on eosinophils, airway hyper-responsiveness, and the late asthmatic response. Lancet. 2000;**356**(9248):2144-2148. DOI: 10.1016/s0140-6736(00)03496-6

[9] Castro M, Zangrilli J, Wechsler ME. Corrections. Reslizumab for inadequately controlled asthma with elevated blood eosinophil counts: Results from two multicentre, parallel, double-blind, randomised, placebo-controlled, phase 3 trials. The Lancet Respiratory Medicine. 2015;**3**(4):e15. DOI: 10.1016/S2213-2600(15)00119-8 Epub 2015 Apr 5. Erratum for: Lancet Respir Med. 2015 May;3(5):355-66

[10] Busse WW, Bleecker ER, FitzGerald JM, Ferguson GT, Barker P, Sproule S, et al. BORA study investigators. Long-term safety and efficacy of benralizumab in patients with severe, uncontrolled asthma: 1-year results from the BORA phase 3 extension trial. The Lancet Respiratory Medicine. 2019;7(1):46-59. DOI: 10.1016/S2213-2600(18)30406-5 Epub 2018 Nov 8. Erratum in: Lancet Respir Med. 2019 Jan;7(1):e1

[11] Wenzel S, Castro M, Corren J, Maspero J, Wang L, Zhang B, et al. Dupilumab efficacy and safety in adults with uncontrolled persistent asthma despite use of medium-to-high-dose inhaled corticosteroids plus a long-acting β2 agonist: A randomised double-blind placebo-controlled pivotal phase 2b dose-ranging trial. Lancet. 2016;**388**(10039):31-44. DOI: 10.1016/S0140-6736(16)30307-5 Epub 2016 Apr 27

[12] Oh CK, Leigh R, McLaurin KK, Kim K, Hultquist M, Molfino NA. A randomized, controlled trial to evaluate the effect of an anti-interleukin-9

monoclonal antibody in adults with uncontrolled asthma. Respiratory Research. 2013;**14**(1):93. DOI: 10.1186/1465-9921-14-93

[13] Humbert M, Taillé C, Mala L, Le Gros V, Just J, Molimard M, et al. Omalizumab effectiveness in patients with severe allergic asthma according to blood eosinophil count: The STELLAIR study. The European Respiratory Journal. 2018;**51**(5):1702523. DOI: 10.1183/13993003.02523-2017

[14] Menzies-Gow A, Corren J, Bourdin A, Chupp G, Israel E, Wechsler ME, et al. Tezepelumab in adults and adolescents with severe, uncontrolled asthma. The New England Journal of Medicine. 2021;**384**(19):1800-1809. DOI: 10.1056/NEJMoa2034975

Chapter 2

The Relationship between microRNAs, ILC2s and Th2 Cells

Feidie Li, Chao Wang, Ran Zhao, Yanhua Niu and Xiaoyan Dong

Abstract

Asthma is a common and chronic inflammatory disease. The pathogenic mechanism underlying asthma is complex. Many inflammatory cells have been recognized as involved in asthma, containing lymphocytes (T, B cells), ILC2s, eosinophils, and other types of immune and inflammatory cells. It is well-established that allergen-specific Th2 cells play a central role in developing allergic asthma. In addition, in recent years, increasing studies have found that ILC2s can contribute to the pathogenesis of asthma by promoting the immune response of Th2 and secreting Th2 cytokines. MicroRNAs (MiRNAs and MiRs) is involved in immune inflammation and can induce excessive secretion of Th2 cytokines. The regulation of miRNAs to their targeting genes plays an important role in the development of asthma. This chapter has discussed altered expression and functions of miRNAs in Th2 and ILC2s in asthma, in order to better understand the mechanics of pathogenesis of asthma, and provide potential miRNA diagnostic indicators and therapeutic targets.

Keywords: asthma, Th2, ILC2s, cytokine, miRNAs

1. Introduction

Asthma is characterized by chronic airway inflammation and airway hyperresponsiveness, it is a heterogeneous disease commonly seen in childhood as a chronic airway disorder [1]. The latest prevalence of childhood asthma in the United States is 5.8% [2], while there is a lack of unified and comprehensive epidemiological survey in China, the prevalence of childhood asthma in China in recent years is about 4.90% through meta-analysis [3], which was higher than the prevalence of the Third National Childhood Asthma Epidemiological Survey of Chinese major cities in 2010 [4]. The research documents the association of immunity with the development of asthma, which is currently believed to be an airway inflammatory disease dominated by a Th2 type of immune response. Found throughout the body in cells, tissues, and body fluids, MicroRNAs are noncoding endogenous RNAs of 19 to 25 nucleotides in number, which base-pair with target gene mRNAs to regulate posttranscriptional expression of the target gene by silencing or blocking the target gene. MicroRNAs are nonspecific and can simultaneously regulate several target genes to fulfill biological roles [5–7]. Their involvement in asthma development has been proven, among others, through the promotion of T cell differentiation toward Th2, the increase of Th2 cytokines, and the decrease of Th1 cytokine secretion [8–11].

Recent studies have highlighted the importance of type 2 innate lymphocytes (ILC2s) in the development of asthma [12, 13]. ILC2s are primarily generated from common lymphoid progenitors (CLPs) in bone marrow, where their maturation proceeds and contributes to intrinsic immunity and tissue repair. It is generally assumed that Th2 cells are the primary source of type 2 cytokines. In contrast, more studies have surfaced that ILC2s can also be a significant early contributor to type 2 cytokines and that such cells can be critical in both the initiation and effector phases of type 2 immunity. ILC2s trigger both the innate response to allergic inflammatory responses and the immune response to adaptive Th2 [14–16]. Experimental stimulation of ILC2s-deficient mice with allergens revealed that the mice did not produce a solid allergic inflammatory response in the lungs and that Th2 cell differentiation was impaired; however, the impaired Th2 cell differentiation was rescued by ILC2 transplantation [15]. Therefore, ILC2s are essential for Th2 cell-mediated allergic lung inflammation and can induce the differentiation of CD4+ T cells into Th2 cells. Furthermore, ILC2s and Th2 cells interact reciprocally during the type 2 immune response, with either the interaction of co-stimulatory molecules or in a direct cell–cell contact-dependent manner through soluble mediators, such as cytokines [17, 18]. In response to the Th2 polarizing cytokines IL-25 and IL-33, ILC2s rely on transcription factors, such as RORα and GATA3, to differentiate and mature [19, 20]. Similarly, n response to IL-4, Th2 cells also depend on transcription factors, such as GATA3, for differentiation and maturation. After the activation of both ILC2s and TH2, a significant amount of Th2 cytokines, IL-4, IL-5, and IL-13 would be produced of which IL-25 is constitutively expressed by clustered cells in the intestine and remains essential for ILC2s to remain stable, IL-25 induces IL-13 production by ILC2s, and IL-13 production by ILC2s and/or Th2 cells may conversely promote differentiation and expansion of clustered cells, creating positive feedback [15, 21, 22]. MiRNAs are increasingly known to regulate the activation of ILC2s and Th2 and Th2-related inflammatory factor production, leading to their involvement in the pathogenesis of asthma. Below is an overview of how miRNAs are involved in asthma development by mediating Th2 and ILC2s.

1.1 Relation between MiRNAs and Th2 differentiation and homeostasis

Th1 and Th2 are in relative homeostasis under normal physiological conditions, whereas an imbalance in the Th1/Th2 ratio and excessive secretion of Th2 cytokines contribute to the pathogenesis of allergic asthma. Most studies have documented that miRNAs are abnormally expressed and are strongly associated with disorders of the Th1/Th2 immune response in asthma [9, 10, 23, 24]. Up or down-regulation of miRNAs can lead to increased secretion of Th2 cytokines or decreased secretion of Th1 cytokines. Up-regulated miRNAs in asthma include miR-21, miR-126, miR-221-3p [25], and miR-3162-3p [26]. Up-regulated miRNAs, including miR-451, miR-1165, miR-29b [27], and miR-135a [28], increased Th2 cytokine secretion include miR-146. As miRNAs can affect T cell differentiation, activation, and eosinophilic mast cell activation in allergic diseases, they could be used as a potential means to reduce Th2 inflammation from the altered genetic level and as noninvasive biomarkers for early prediction of asthma development. Of the many publications on how miRNAs regulate Th2 cells, a few of the most extensive studies are presented below.

1.2 MiR-155

MiR-155 is an indispensable miRNA for functioning dendritic cells, T cells, B cells, and other immune cells. In the past, much attention has been focused on miR-155's involvement in pro-inflammation and Th1 immunity, and it is labeled as a "Th2 inhibitor" [29]. When compared to WT mice, for example, miR-155(−/−) mice showed significantly lower numbers of inflammatory cells in alveolar lavage fluid, which compromised the initiation of Th2 responses and reduced airway inflammation [8]. With further studies, however, miR-155 shows an integral contribution to allergic asthma. Therefore, in patients with asthma, there is decreased expression of miR-155 in peripheral blood CD4+ T cells, notably in severe asthma [30], meaning it is strongly associated with asthma severity, which may be achieved by directly targeting the IL-13 pathway suggesting that a strong correlation between miR-155 and asthma severity exists, which is probably attained by directly targeting the IL-13 pathway [31]. Compared to WT mice, miR-155-deficient mice have significantly reduced eosinophil content in alveolar lavage fluid after allergen stimulation [32], demonstrating that Mir-155 may gather more eosinophils during airway inflammation. In a similar vein, Kim constructed mouse models of miR-155 deficiency in T cells and identified lower levels of Th2 cytokines in alveolar lavage fluid and lower mucus secretion in the experimental group compared to the control group [33]. These findings recommend that miR-155 from T cells is essential for Th2 allergic airway inflammation as a crucial serological biomarker for asthma diagnosis and severity.

1.3 MiR-21

Statistical studies of clinical data have found significantly higher levels of miR-21-3p and miR-487b-3p expression among the sera of children in the acute phase of food allergic reactions [34], presumably due to the targeted binding of lL-12 and miR-21-3p, which by down-regulating the former, could promote th2 inflammatory responses. Similarly, studies in an asthma rat model experiment revealed that miR-21-5p expression was significantly up-regulated, mainly in alveolar macrophages. MiR-21-5p produced by macrophages was confirmed by *in vitro* experiments to be targeted by the TGF-β1/Smad-signaling circuit to Smad7 after translocation to the airway epithelium for promoting EMT (epithelial-mesenchymal transition) [35], thereby enhancing airway remodeling leading to the development of asthma. Zhou demonstrated the involvement of mast cells in asthma development in an asthma model, where miR-21 was present in derived EV and could exacerbate the airway inflammatory response in mice via the DDAH1/Wnt/β-catenin axis [36]. Furthermore, a significant reduction in Th2 cytokine expression, an increase in IL-12 and IFN-γ secretion, and a reduction in cup cells in lung tissue were observed in miR-21-deficient asthmatic mice [37], which in turn attenuated airway inflammation as well as remodeling. From the above, miR-21 can be involved in the development and progression of asthma by promoting Th2 differentiation and airway remodeling through various inflammatory response signaling pathways. It can serve as a potential biomarker for allergic reactions.

1.4 let-7 family

The let-7 family was found as a second microRNA, down-regulated in various tumors and also referred to as a tumor suppressor. However, there is some controversy about the role of let-7miRNAs in asthma. IL-13, a critical Th2 cytokine, was also a direct target of let-7 microRNAs, some of which were suggested to play an anti-inflammatory role in the immune response. Manis agreed that let-7miRNAs possessed an anti-inflammatory action and concluded that let-7miRNAs reduced the inflammatory response by targeting the IL-13 3'UTR site, thereby lowering IL-13 levels through *ex vivo* experiments in asthma models [38]. Instead, Polikepahad has found a pro-inflammatory effect of let-7 in a mouse model of asthma [39], which may be associated with differences in experimental methods, making it even keener for further study by those to follow. In addition, it has been found that let-7 inhibitors can enhance the effect of airway smooth muscle on β2-receptor agonists by reducing β2-receptors downregulateion [40], which is more effective in asthma control.

1.5 MiR-126

The relative levels of miR-126 in the peripheral blood of children with asthma were found to be both elevated and significantly correlated with the severity of the disease and also negatively correlated with IFN-γ levels, which has great potential for diagnosis, especially in severe asthma, with an AUC of 0.909 [41], as one of the diagnostic biomarkers for asthma. The up-regulated levels of miR-126 were positively correlated with the severity of lung function [42], which may be associated with IL-13 [41]. But they have higher small airway reversibility [43]. Concerning animal experiments, Mattes found in an ovalbumin (OVA)-induced asthma model that miR-126 blockade led to enhanced expression of POU structural domain class 2 associated factor 1, one that activates the transcription factor PU.1, which alters TH2 cell function by negatively regulating GATA3 expression [44]. GATA3 may facilitate Th0 to Th2 differentiation. During the construction of the chronic airway inflammation model, the expression of multiple miRNAs, especially miR-126, increased in the airway wall early in the model establishment, and when administered with miR-126 antagonists, inhibited airway eosinophil recruitment. In contrast, later in the model construction, miR-126 expression decreased, and continued administration of miR-126 antagonists affected long-term chronic inflammation of the airway walls with little change [45]. These results indicate that miR-126 plays a significant role early in pathological evolution and that early intervention should be of little clinical significance if it reaches a terminal stage.

1.6 Other related miRNAs

Analysis of clinical data identified that children with asthma presented with reduced levels of miR-34a, miR-92b, and miR-210 secretion from airway epithelial extracellular vesicle (EV), while the decline may enable DCs to polarize Th2 cells, giving rise to the asthma phenotype [46]. The extraction of lymphocytes from asthmatic children yielded significantly lower levels of miR-451a than baseline, miRNA-451a with an FC of 4.6 and a p-value of 0.008 (asthma vs. control), and down-regulation of miR-451a was observed when CD4+ T cells were placed in Th2 differentiation medium and ETS1 upregulation, leading to the evidence that miRNA-451 inhibits Th2 differentiation by downregulating EST1 [47]. Furthermore, a significant reduction in type 2 allergic lung inflammation was observed in asthma model mice with upregulation of miR-1165-3p in mouse lung tissue, suggesting that miR-1165-3p could inhibit Th2 differentiation, which was achieved by directly targeting IL-13 and PPM1A [48]. In addition, miR-29b upregulation in an asthma model can modify the Th1/Th2 balance by inhibiting ICOS expression, thereby attenuating eosinophil recruitment in airway epithelial cells [49]. MiRNAs have a profound impact on the regulation of allergic inflammation and are expected to become biomarkers for allergic diseases, such as asthma, as well as important therapeutic targets in the future. MiRNAs with a profound impact on the regulation of allergic inflammation are expected to be biomarkers for allergic diseases, such as asthma, and may likewise be a valuable therapeutic target in the future.

2. MicroRNAs and ILC2s

Derived from typical lymph-like progenitor cells in the bone marrow and expressed in tissues, such as the lung, ILC2s are considered the innate counterpart of Th2 cells and have a collaborative role in the pathogenesis of allergic diseases. Belonging to the innate immune system, ILC2s do not articulate rearranged specific antigen receptors, but their activation is mainly controlled by epithelial cytokines, such as TSLP, IL-25, and IL-33. Among these, IL-33 and IL-25 are potent activators of ILC2. ILC2s can be characterized by the generation of type 2 cytokines (IL-13, IL-4, and IL-5) and the expression of GATA-3 transcription factors. Located strategically in the airway mucosa, ILC2 can be critical for patrolling the airway, enrolling other immune system cells, and activating resident cells in response to pathogenic injury or tissue damage [50]. Consequently, ILC2s have been studied for their development, proliferation, and expression. The study of the underlying mechanisms of ILC2 is of current interest; however, extensive research on ILC2s has in recent years yielded the conclusion that it is ILC2s that act as the significant secretory drivers of allergic inflammation and contribute significantly to airway disease models [51]. Therefore, the following section will describe the effects of various miRNAs, including miR-155, miR-1146, and miR-206, on ILC2s, as an increasing amount of research has been devoted to ILC2s.

2.1 MiR-155

There is no doubt that the development of the immune system, the maturation and differentiation of immune cells, and the stability of their function are inseparable from the involvement of miR-155, which participates in the modulation of the Th2 immune response in eosinophilic airway inflammation. Analyzing the nasal mucosa and peripheral blood collected from allergic rhinitis (AR) patients, Zhu revealed that the miR-155, IL-25, and IL-33 in nasal mucosa exceeded those in controls, as did ILC2s in blood, all of which had statistical significance. Later, a mouse model of LAR was built to validate this idea and concluded that miR-155 was indispensable in the proliferation and activation of ILC2s induced by IL-33 [52]. In other words, overexpression of miR-155 facilitates the overexpression of ILC2s, triggering many type 2 cytokines and a series of allergic phenotypes. The same conclusion came from Wan's study of AR mouse models, where miR-155 not only promoted Th2 differentiation but also increased the number of ILC2s [53]. With the mouse model of asthma, however, Martin concluded that miR-155 could protect ILC2 from apoptosis in a way that boosted the type 2 immune response, given the small effect of miR-155 on ILC2 cell proliferation as well as cytokines [54]. Indeed, they have mutual recognition of miR-155 as required for ILC2s to respond to IL-33 amplification [55]. The proliferation in the absence of miR-155 can be complex for those ILC2s, albeit through intrinsic mechanisms that need further investigation. Nevertheless, one thing is sure, miR-155 is instrumental in the proliferation, activation, and functional stability of ILC2s.

2.2 MiR-146

The anti-inflammatory properties of MiR-146a can be seen in human bronchial epithelial cells during rhinovirus infection and allergic inflammation and in the airways of mice [56]. Targeting miR-146 may be a novel strategy for the treatment of allergic asthma. In mouse models of asthma, treatment of IL-33-activated ILC2s with miR-146a decreased the ability of ILC2s to secrete cytokines, whereas no effects were observed in IL-25-activated ILC2s. Meanwhile, the ability of ILC2 to secrete IL-13 and IL-5 was increased after miR-146a inhibitor treatment, and the results after miR-146 administration showed no significant change in IL-33 and IL-25 expression levels in mice [57, 58]. Thus, miR-146a may reduce the airway inflammatory response in asthma by blocking the IL-33 pathway, by inhibiting IRAK1 and TRAF6, downstream molecules of ST2 signal pathway, to negatively regulate IL-33/ST2-activated ILC2 to inhibit asthma [59]. But a pathway other than IL-25 cannot be excluded. Consequently, we conclude that miR-146a could be one of the most effective therapeutic options for the anti-inflammatory treatment of asthma.

2.3 Other ILC2s

According to Zhang, T2-type asthmatics showed lower airway epithelial miR-206 than normal subjects, including higher levels in type 2 hyper asthmatics than in type 2 hypo asthmatics. As a result, an animal model is built to suggest that higher miR-206 in type 2 hyper asthma can reduce CD39, an ATP degrading ectonucleotidase and a target of miR-206, whose accumulation exacerbates asthma [60]. Many cells can secrete EVs extracted from the supernatant of human mast cells (MC). Their miRNA profiling shows that miR103a-3p is markedly up-regulated and enhances IL-5 production by ILC2s after coculture with human ILC2s [61] through methylation of GATA3 arginine residues. While ICAM-1 appears to be essential for ILC2 development and function, it has been found in AR patients and animal models that overexpression of miR-150-5p can decrease ICAM-1 expression, whereas a decrease in ICAM-1 can led to a downregulation of GATA3 levels, which can, in turn, inhibit the function of ILC2s from alleviating allergic symptoms [62]. The results of an *in vivo* study in a mouse model of AR showed that miR-375 enhanced the function of ILC2s by regulating TSLP [63], providing a potential therapeutic target for AR. The miR-17 ~ 92 gene cluster Th2 secretes related cytokines, of which miR-19a takes a significant role. By constructing a mouse model of asthma, miR-19a promoted the activation and proliferation of ILC2s, thereby increasing the secretion of IL-13 and IL-5 [51]. Roberts' study showed a biased development of ILC2s progenitors in the bone marrow of mir142−/− mice compared to wild-type mice, with a dysregulated proliferative effect of ILC2s [64]. These findings indicate that miR-142 maintains the homeostasis of ILC2s in tissues, similar to miR-155 and miR-19. With the increasing prominence of ILC2s in allergic diseases as a top research priority related to the pathogenesis of asthma to date, it is believed that further studies will undoubtedly identify additional relationships between miRNAs and ILC2s.

3. The relationship between microRNAs, ILC2s, and Th2 cells

Asthma is a complex disease engaged by multiple mechanisms on a nonhomogeneous basis. Asthma has variable conditions in terms of clinical presentation (phenotype) and different pathophysiological mechanisms (endotype) [65]. An imbalance in the Th1/Th2 ratio and hypersecretion of Th2 cytokines are currently thought pivotal in the pathogenesis of allergic asthma. Cells that produce Th2-type cytokines include type 2 helper T cells (Th2), follicular helper T cells (TFH), basophils, mast cells, and type 2 innate lymphoid-like cells (ILC2s). ILC2s and Th2 cells can induce type 2 immunopathology by releasing type 2 effector cytokines [66]. As a result, ILC2s offer a primary source of early intrinsic cells driving the classical type 2 cytokines in eosinophilic inflammation. Participating as regulators of immunity by coordinating multiple target genes in multiple cells, MiRNAs can modulate Th2 cell differentiation, Th1/Th2 balance, and promote type 2 immune responses, and thus participate in the development and progression of asthma. ILC2s are critical initiators of allergic inflammation. They all participate in asthma onset and development. Many miRNAs mentioned above are involved in Th2 cell responses and ILC2s reactions, contributing to more or less the development of allergic diseases. Priti, who compared the miRNAs transcriptomes of ILC2s and Th2 cells in lung tissue, concluded that miRNAs expression is necessary to maintain ILC2 homeostasis *in vivo*, which can be mediated by participating in the regulation of overlapping but not identical target genes of innate and adaptive immune cells to achieve certain expected biological outcomes that can contribute to the development of allergic disease [51]. Therefore, we might also consider that specific miRNAs affect both Th2 and ILC2s through common pathways, exacerbating or contributing to certain allergic diseases, such as asthma. A common link between MicroRNAs, ILC2s, and Th2 remains to be further investigated.

Author details

Feidie Li*, Chao Wang, Ran Zhao, Yanhua Niu and Xiaoyan Dong
Department of Respiratory Medicine, Shanghai Children's Hospital, Shanghai Jiao Tong University School of Medicine, Shanghai, China

*Address all correspondence to: feidie188@163.com

IntechOpen

© 2022 The Author(s). Licensee IntechOpen. This chapter is distributed under the terms of the Creative Commons Attribution License (http://creativecommons.org/licenses/by/3.0), which permits unrestricted use, distribution, and reproduction in any medium, provided the original work is properly cited. (cc) BY

References

[1] Guideline for the diagnosis and optimal management of asthma in children (2016). Zhonghua Er Ke Za Zhi. 2016;**54**(3):167-181

[2] CDC Asthma Stats Reports and Publications. 2022; Available from: https://www.cdc.gov/asthma/most_recent_national_asthma_data.htm

[3] Shu Z, Jia H, Yali L, et al. Prevalence and risk factors of childhood asthma in China: A Meta-analysis. International Journal of Epidemiology and Infectious Diseases. 2020;**03**:253-259

[4] Third nationwide survey of childhood asthma in urban areas of China. Zhonghua Er Ke Za Zhi. 2013;**51**(10):729-735

[5] Carthew RW, Sontheimer EJ. Origins and mechanisms of miRNAs and siRNAs. Cell. 2009;**136**(4):642-655

[6] Mohr AM, Mott JL. Overview of microRNA biology. Seminars in Liver Disease. 2015;**35**(1):3-11

[7] Sayed D, Abdellatif M. MicroRNAs in development and disease. Physiological Reviews. 2011;**91**(3):827-887

[8] Zech A, Ayata CK, Pankratz F, et al. MicroRNA-155 modulates P2R signaling and Th2 priming of dendritic cells during allergic airway inflammation in mice. Allergy. 2015;**70**(9):1121-1129

[9] Feng MJ, Shi F, Qiu C, et al. MicroRNA-181a, −146a and -146b in spleen CD4+ T lymphocytes play proinflammatory roles in a murine model of asthma [J]. International Immunopharmacology. 2012;**13**(3):347-353

[10] Suojalehto H, Lindström I, Majuri ML, et al. Altered microRNA expression of nasal mucosa in long-term asthma and allergic rhinitis [J]. International Archives of Allergy and Immunology. 2014;**163**(3):168-178

[11] Yu Y, Wang L, Gu G. The correlation between Runx3 and bronchial asthma. Clinica Chimica Acta. 2018;**487**:75-79

[12] Maggi L, Mazzoni A, Capone M, et al. The dual function of ILC2: From host protection to pathogenic players in type 2 asthma. Molecular Aspects of Medicine. 2021;**80**:100981

[13] Boonpiyathad T, Sözener ZC, Satitsuksanoa P, et al. Immunologic mechanisms in asthma. Seminars in Immunology. 2019;**46**:101333

[14] Martinez-Gonzalez I, Steer CA, Takei F. Lung ILC2s link innate and adaptive responses in allergic inflammation. Trends in Immunology. 2015;**36**(3):189-195

[15] Halim TY, Steer CA, Mathä L, et al. Group 2 innate lymphoid cells are critical for the initiation of adaptive T helper 2 cell-mediated allergic lung inflammation. Immunity. 2014;**40**(3):425-435

[16] Neill DR, Wong SH, Bellosi A, et al. Nuocytes represent a new innate effector leukocyte that mediates type-2 immunity. Nature. 2010;**464**(7293):1367-1370

[17] Sonnenberg GF, Hepworth MR. Functional interactions between innate lymphoid cells and adaptive immunity. Nature Reviews. Immunology. 2019;**19**(10):599-613

[18] Symowski C, Voehringer D. Interactions between innate lymphoid

cells and cells of the innate and adaptive immune system. Frontiers in Immunology. 2017;**8**:1422

[19] Kabata H, Moro K, Koyasu S. The group 2 innate lymphoid cell (ILC2) regulatory network and its underlying mechanisms [J]. Immunological Reviews. 2018;**286**(1):37-52

[20] Martinez-Gonzalez I, Ghaedi M, Steer CA, et al. ILC2 memory: Recollection of previous activation. Immunological Reviews. 2018;**283**(1):41-53

[21] Drake LY, Iijima K, Kita H. Group 2 innate lymphoid cells and CD4+ T cells cooperate to mediate type 2 immune response in mice. Allergy. 2014;**69**(10):1300-1307

[22] Oeser K, Schwartz C, Voehringer D. Conditional IL-4/IL-13-deficient mice reveal a critical role of innate immune cells for protective immunity against gastrointestinal helminths. Mucosal Immunology. 2015;**8**(3):672-682

[23] Hammad H, Lambrecht BN. The basic immunology of asthma. Cell. 2021;**184**(6):1469-1485

[24] Simpson LJ, Patel S, Bhakta NR, et al. A microRNA upregulated in asthma airway T cells promotes TH2 cytokine production. Nature Immunology. 2014;**15**(12):1162-1170

[25] Dong W, Lu W. Effect of long non-coding RNA NEAT1 in asthmatic inflammation and cell barrier damage by regulating miR-221-3. The Chinese Journal of Clinical Pharmacology. 2022;**38**(6):495-498

[26] Juman L. Effects of miR-3162-3p on lung inflammation and autophagy in asthmatic mouse. 2020

[27] Yue-Yue W, Wei J, Zheng-Rong C, et al. Effect of macrophage polarization regulated by miR-29b, B7-H3 on CD4+T cell differentiation in asthma. Journal of Hainan Medical University. 2021;**27**(7):506-512

[28] Huang XP, Qin CY, Gao YM. miR-135a inhibits airway inflammatory response in asthmatic mice via regulating JAK/STAT signaling pathway. Brazilian Journal of Medical and Biological Research. 2021;**54**(3):e10023

[29] Banerjee A, Schambach F, Dejong CS, et al. Micro-RNA-155 inhibits IFN-gamma signaling in CD4+ T cells [J]. European Journal of Immunology. 2010;**40**(1):225-231

[30] Zhang YY, Zhong M, Zhang MY, et al. Expression and clinical significance of miR-155 in peripheral blood CD4(+);T cells of patients with allergic asthma. Xi Bao Yu Fen Zi Mian Yi Xue Za Zhi. 2012;**28**(5):540-543

[31] Martinez-Nunez RT, Louafi F, Sanchez-Elsner T. The interleukin 13 (IL-13) pathway in human macrophages is modulated by microRNA-155 via direct targeting of interleukin 13 receptor alpha1 (IL13Ralpha1). The Journal of Biological Chemistry. 2011;**286**(3):1786-1794

[32] Malmhäll C, Alawieh S, Lu Y, et al. MicroRNA-155 is essential for T(H)2-mediated allergen-induced eosinophilic inflammation in the lung. Journal of Allergy and Clinical Immunology. 2014;**133**(5):1429-1438

[33] Kim HJ, Park SO, Byeon HW, et al. T cell-intrinsic miR-155 is required for Th2 and Th17-biased responses in acute and chronic airway inflammation by targeting several different transcription factors. Immunology. 2022:e13477

[34] Nuñez-Borque E, Fernandez-Bravo S, Rodriguez Del Rio P, et al. Increased miR-21-3p and miR-487b-3p serum levels during anaphylactic reaction in food allergic children. Pediatric Allergy and Immunology. 2021;**32**(6):1296-1306

[35] Li X, Yang N, Cheng Q, et al. MiR-21-5p in macrophage-derived exosomes targets Smad7 to promote epithelial mesenchymal transition of airway epithelial cells. Journal of Asthma and Allergy. 2021;**14**:513-524

[36] Zou Y, Zhou Q, Zhang Y. MicroRNA-21 released from mast cells-derived extracellular vesicles drives asthma in mice by potentiating airway inflammation and oxidative stress. American Journal of Translational Research. 2021;**13**(7):7475-7491

[37] Lee HY, Hur J, Kang JY, et al. MicroRNA-21 inhibition suppresses alveolar M2 macrophages in an ovalbumin-induced allergic asthma mice model. Allergy Asthma Immunological Research. 2021;**13**(2):312-329

[38] Kumar M, Ahmad T, Sharma A, et al. Let-7 microRNA-mediated regulation of IL-13 and allergic airway inflammation [J]. The Journal of Allergy and Clinical Immunology. 2011;**128**(5):1077

[39] Polikepahad S, Knight JM, Naghavi AO, et al. Proinflammatory role for let-7 microRNAS in experimental asthma. The Journal of Biological Chemistry. 2010;**285**(39):30139-30149

[40] Van Den Berge M, Tasena H. Role of microRNAs and exosomes in asthma. Current Opinion in Pulmonary Medicine. 2019;**25**(1):87-93

[41] Tian M, Ji Y, Wang T, et al. Changes in circulating microRNA-126 levels are associated with immune imbalance in children with acute asthma. International Journal of Immunopathology and Pharmacology. 2018;**32**:205

[42] Tingshi W. The value of miR-126 in evaluating the severity of patients with bronchial asthma. Laboratory Medicine and Clinic. 2017;**14**(15):2233-2235

[43] Mendes FC, Paciência I, Ferreira AC, et al. Development and validation of exhaled breath condensate microRNAs to identify and endotype asthma in children. PLoS One. 2019;**14**(11):e0224983

[44] Mattes J, Collison A, Plank M, et al. Antagonism of microRNA-126 suppresses the effector function of TH2 cells and the development of allergic airways disease. Proceedings of the National Academy of Sciences of the United States of America. 2009;**106**(44):18704-18709

[45] Collison A, Herbert C, Siegle JS, et al. Altered expression of microRNA in the airway wall in chronic asthma: miR-126 as a potential therapeutic target. BMC Pulmonary Medicine. 2011;**11**:29

[46] Bartel S, la Grutta S, Cilluffo G, et al. Human airway epithelial extracellular vesicle miRNA signature is altered upon asthma development. Allergy. 2020;**75**(2):346-356

[47] Wang T, Zhou Q, Shang Y. Downregulation of miRNA-451a promotes the differentiation of CD4+ T cells towards Th2 cells by upregulating ETS1 in childhood asthma. Journal of Innate Immunity. 2021;**13**(1):38-48

[48] Wang Z, Ji N, Chen Z, et al. MiR-1165-3p suppresses Th2 differentiation via targeting IL-13 and PPM1A in a mouse model of allergic airway inflammation. Allergy Asthma and Immunological Research. 2020;**12**(5):859-876

[49] Yan J, Zhang X, Sun S, et al. miR-29b reverses T helper 1 cells/T helper 2 cells imbalance and alleviates airway eosinophils recruitment in OVA-induced murine asthma by targeting inducible Co-stimulator. International Archives of Allergy and Immunology. 2019;**180**(3):182-194

[50] Diefenbach A, Colonna M, Koyasu S. Development, differentiation, and diversity of innate lymphoid cells. Immunity. 2014;**41**(3):354-365

[51] Singh PB, Pua HH, Happ HC, et al. MicroRNA regulation of type 2 innate lymphoid cell homeostasis and function in allergic inflammation. The Journal of Experimental Medicine. 2017;**214**(12):3627-3643

[52] Zhu YQ, Liao B, Liu YH, et al. MicroRNA-155 plays critical effects on Th2 factors expression and allergic inflammatory response in type-2 innate lymphoid cells in allergic rhinitis. European Review for Medical and Pharmacological Sciences. 2019;**23**(10):4097-4109

[53] Renpeng W. MiR-155 regulates ILC2 of allergic rhinitis mice via C-maf. 2020

[54] Knolle MD, Chin SB, Rana BMJ, et al. MicroRNA-155 protects group 2 innate lymphoid cells from apoptosis to promote Type-2 immunity. Frontiers in Immunology. 2018;**9**:2232

[55] Johansson K, Malmhäll C, Ramos-Ramírez P, et al. MicroRNA-155 is a critical regulator of type 2 innate lymphoid cells and IL-33 signaling in experimental models of allergic airway inflammation. The Journal of Allergy and Clinical Immunology. 2017;**139**(3):1007-16.e9

[56] Laanesoo A, Urgard E, Periyasamy K, et al. Dual role of the miR-146 family in rhinovirus-induced airway inflammation and allergic asthma exacerbation [J]. Clinical and Translational Medicine. 2021;**11**(6):e427

[57] Shugaung H. The role and molecular mechanism of miR-146a in regulating type 2 innate lymphocytes (ILC2s) in asthma. 2019

[58] Han S, Ma C, Bao L, et al. miR-146a mimics attenuate allergic airway inflammation by impacted group 2 innate lymphoid cells in an ovalbumin-induced asthma mouse model. International Archives of Allergy and Immunology. 2018;**177**(4):302-310

[59] Lyu B, Wei Z, Jiang L, et al. MicroRNA-146a negatively regulates IL-33 in activated group 2 innate lymphoid cells by inhibiting IRAK1 and TRAF6. Genes and Immunity. 2020;**21**(1):37-44

[60] Zhang K, Feng Y, Liang Y, et al. Epithelial miR-206 targets CD39/extracellular ATP to upregulate airway IL-25 and TSLP in type 2-high asthma. JCI Insight. 2021;**6**(11)

[61] Toyoshima S, Sakamoto-Sasaki T, Kurosawa Y, et al. miR103a-3p in extracellular vesicles from FcεRI-aggregated human mast cells enhances IL-5 production by group 2 innate lymphoid cells. The Journal of Allergy and Clinical Immunology. 2021;**147**(5):1878-1891

[62] Zhang L, Meng W, Chen X, et al. MiR-150-5p regulates the functions of type 2 innate lymphoid cells via the ICAM-1/p38 MAPK axis in allergic rhinitis. Molecular and Cellular Biochemistry. 2022;**477**(4):1009-1022

[63] Luo X, Zeng Q, Yan S, et al. MicroRNA-375-mediated regulation of ILC2 cells through TSLP in allergic

rhinitis. World Allergy Organization Journal. 2020;**13**(8):100451

[64] Roberts LB, Jowett GM, Read E, et al. MicroRNA-142 critically regulates group 2 innate lymphoid cell homeostasis and function. Journal of Immunology. 2021;**206**(11):2725-2739

[65] Andrea M, Susanna B, Francesca N, et al. The emerging role of type 2 inflammation in asthma. Expert Review of Clinical Immunology. 2021;**17**(1):63-71

[66] Gurram RK, Zhu J. Orchestration between ILC2s and Th2 cells in shaping type 2 immune responses. Cellular & Molecular Immunology. 2019;**16**(3):225-235

Chapter 3

The Blood Biomarkers of Asthma

Chen Hao, Cui Yubao and Zhu Rongfei

Abstract

Asthma was a chronic inflammatory airway disease which characterized by complex pathogenesis, various clinical manifestations and severity. Blood biomarkers have been used to evaluate the severity of the disease, predict the efficacy and prognosis. Currently, some incredible progress in most of the research on biomarkers for asthma have achieved, including cell, antibodies, cytokines, chemokines, proteins and non-coding RNAs. We reviewed the application of these biomarkers in diagnosis, treatment, prognosis monitoring and phenotypic identification of asthma, in order to improve clinicians' understanding of asthma biomarkers.

Keywords: biomarker, asthma, cell, antibodies, cytokines, chemokines, proteins, non-coding RNAs

1. Introduction

Asthma was a chronic inflammatory airway disease which characterized by complex pathogenesis, various clinical manifestations and severity. With an increasing prevalence, asthma affecting an estimated 358 million people worldwide [1]. According to the recent epidemiological data in China, there were 45.7 million adult patients with asthma and the total prevalence rate was 4.2% [2]. The cumulative prevalence among children under 14 years of age was 3.02% [3]. The high prevalence and different clinical manifestations lead to various treatment of asthma. Therefore, it was very important to determine the classification and specific markers for the management of asthma.

Francisaca et al. have proposed to classify asthma phenotypes into allergic asthma, eosinophilic asthma, obese asthma, persistent asthma, symptomatic asthma, positive bronchial provocation test with asthma symptoms, positive bronchial provocation test with no asthma symptoms, and negative bronchial provocation test with asthma symptoms [4]. This classification method mainly focuses on the presentation of symptoms and does not guide the precise treatment of asthma patients. Identifying the phenotype of asthma according to the molecular mechanism can solve this problem to a certain extent.

Asthma can be classified into T2 and non-T2 asthma according to the molecular mechanism of airway inflammation. The former was mainly composed of eosinophils (EOS), mast cell (MC), dendritic cells (DC), and Type 2 innate lymphoid cells (ILC2), which secrete immunoglobulin E (IgE), Interleukin-4 (IL-4), IL-5, IL-13, IL-33, prostaglandin D2, thymic stromal lymphopoietin (TSLP) and other antibodies and inflammatory factors. Non-T2 asthma was involved in the secretion of cytokines such as IL-1, IL-6, IL-17, CXCL-1 and 8, interferon-γ (IFN-γ), and tumor necrosis factor (TNF)-α by inflammatory cells such as neutrophils (NEU) [5]. A number of biomarkers have been identified in broncho alveolar lavage (BAL), peripheral blood, induced sputum, and bronchial biopsy tissue and etc. According to the pathogenesis of different asthma phenotypes, among these samples, peripheral blood can be easily obtained in clinic practice. Thus, we investigate potential biomarkers in peripheral blood for asthma patients, in order to enhance the management and treatment of asthma.

2. Blood biomarkers of asthma

2.1 Cellular biomarkers

EOS in peripheral blood were considered as an important biomarker for asthma, and can predict the treatment response [6]. A small prospective cohort study of hospitalized infants with asthma demonstrated that elevated EOS in convalescence can predict an increased risk of asthma in the future [7, 8] Neutrophils (NEU) in peripheral blood can assess asthma control and prognosis, the counts of NEU over 5000/ul means that asthma symptoms were poorly controlled and likely to get worse [9]. Basophils contains cytoplasmic secretory granules, and was consisted by proteoglycans and histamine [10]. Basophil activation test (BAT) was a useful method for marking CD63 and CD203c, which were the most common surface markers of basophil activation. The detection of CD63 and CD203c implied that basophil degranulation and may led to histamine release, which provide crucial information for the diagnosis of allergic asthma [11].

Mast cell (MC) also played an important role in allergic inflammation. A study suggested that interactions between mast cells and airway smooth muscle cells were critical for the development of the disordered airway physiology in asthma [12]. Therefore, mast cell activation test can be used as a diagnostic method of asthma.

Innate lymphoid cells (ILC), which was different from T cells and B cells, are located on the mucosal surface of the intestine and played an important role in enhancing the immune response, maintaining mucosal integrity and promoting the formation of lymphoid organs. According to the cytokine expression profile, ILC can be divided into three groups: ILC1, ILC2 and ILC3, among which ILC2 can produce a large number of T2 cytokines, such as IL-5 and IL-13 [13], which can promote EOS and airway hyperresponsiveness (AHR), led to exacerbating the symptoms of asthma. The level of activated ILC2s in blood, bronchoalveolar lavage fluid (BALF), and sputum of asthmatic patients were increasing compared with healthy controls [14]. Thus, ILC2 can be regard as an important biomarker for the assessment of asthma.

T helper (Th2) and non Th2 were phenotypes of asthma and have been determined by CD4+T cells [15]. Th2 asthma was characterized by elevated EOS and high levels of interleukin (IL)-4, IL-5 and IL-13 [16]. In contrast, non Th2 asthma was characterized by NEU infiltration and high levels of IFN-γ and IL-17 [15]. Since the progression pattern and treatment plan of asthma depend on the differentiation of CD4+T cells, clarifying the biological role of CD4+T cells in the pathogenesis of asthma was very important to develop effective treatment and predict the prognosis of asthma patients [17].

Forkhead box P3 (Foxp3)+ regulatory T (Treg) cells were a special subgroup of CD4+T cells, which played a key role in maintaining immune tolerance and inhibiting immune response to antigens [18]. In patients with severe asthma, the number of Treg cells in blood, BALF and sputum was decreased [19, 20], which concluded that Treg cells can be used to assess asthma severity.

Macrophages were account for about 70% of the immune cells in the asllergic asthma, and played an important role in airway inflammation [20]. A study has shown that the impaired function of alveolar macrophages always be presented in children with poorly controlled asthma which were, characterized by decreased phagocytosis and increased apoptosis [21]. Therefore, macrophages also play an important role in assessment of asthma administration.

2.2 Antibody biomarkers

Mucosal IgA neutralizes bacteria and viruses by interfering with epithelial adhesion and improving the characteristics of mucus capture and antigen removal [22]. One report have shown that infants with low IgA levels have more common asthma and more severe allergic symptoms. In addition, infants born to allergic parents were more prone to deficiency of salivary IgA [23]. Another report shows that serum IgA levels in adult patients with asthma are associated with asthma severity [24]. Therefore, IgA level has certain guiding significance for the severity of asthma symptoms.

The amount of total IgE (tIgE) in serum and the presence of allergen-specific IgE(sIgE) antibodies are important biomarkers to assess the phenotype and symptoms of asthma patients. The level of sIgE in serum may also be helpful to predict persistent wheezing. Furthermore, tIgE was associated with asthma and can be considered as a supplementary indicator for the severity of asthma [25]. One study investigated that in the HDM sensitized children, the ratio of sIgG to sIgE in asthma children was significantly lower than that of non-asthma children, and was the lowest among the children with the most severe asthmatic symptoms, which speculated that sIgG may play a certain inhibitory role in the pathogenesis of asthma [26]. Thus, sIgG/sIgE has been used as a biomarker for more accurate evaluation of asthma than single sIgE.

2.3 Cytokine markers

Allergic asthma was driven by T-helper type 2 (Th2) cells, inducing the production of inflammatory cytokines such as IL-4, IL-5 and IL-13. IL-4 and IL-13 are key drivers of a variety of atopic diseases [27]. In addition to Th2 cells, other lymphocytes include γδT cell subsets, natural killer T (NKT) cells, T follicular helper cells (Tfh) cells and type 2 innate lymphoid cells (ILC2s) can also produce IL-4 and/or IL-13 [28]. IL-4 was a differentiation factor that polarizes naive CD4+T cells to Th2 phenotype [29]. It was essential in inducing local Th2 response and the development of pulmonary eosinophilic inflammation [30], but didn't have direct effect on mucus production [31].

IL-5 can increase expression of C-C chemokine receptor 3 (CCR3) by mature EOS [32], it was also conducive to the recruitment and activation of EOS in asthma patients [33]. Although the activation of Th2 cells in allergic asthma lead to the increase of some cytokines, such as IL-13, IL-4, IL-5, and granulocyte-macrophage colony-stimulating factor (GM-CSF) [34], the predominant cytokine associated with antigen-induced eosinophilic inflammation still was IL-5 [35]. In brief, IL-5 palyed an important role in the evaluation of eosinophilic inflammation in asthma.

IL-13 can induce B cells to synthesize IgG4 and IgE, which provided pivotal signal in allergic disease [36]. As aT2 inflammatory cytokins, IL-13 can be produced by CD4+T, EOS, MC, basophils, and NKT [37]. IL-13 had various roles in asthma, for example, it can switched antibody synthesis of plasma cell and produced IgE, and promoted the migration of EOS to the lungs. Because of the EOS synthesis and the up-regulation of adhesion molecules bound to EOS, goblet cell proliferation and mucus production would increased, which lead to increased sputum and AHR [38].

Asthma patients have a higher levels of serum IL-4, IL-5 and IL-13 compared with healthy controls these cytokines were also increased in acute asthma [39]. A clinical study has shown that blocking both IL-4 and IL-13 signaling can significantly reduce the exacerbation of severe asthma [40], and after anti-IL-5 treatment, 83% of patients with severe asthma had a favorable responses [41].

CD4+T cells, particularly activated Th2 cells, have been found to represent a major cellular source for IL-31 [42]. Polymorphisms in IL-31 is associated with IgE production in asthma patients [43]. at the same time, IL-31 promoted the occurrence of chemokines and pro-inflammatory cytokines in human bronchial epithelial cells (HBECs), and could lead to a Th2-dominant inflammation in asthma [44]. The levels of IL-31 in serum and BALF were increased in asthma patients and IL-31 also was positively correlated with Th2 cytokines (IL-5, IL-13, TSLP) and the severity of asthma [45].

Th17 related cytokines such as IL-17A, IL-17F, IL-21 and IL-22 were secreted by Th17 cells. In the mice model of allergic asthma, the impairment of IL-17R signal delayed the recruitment of neutrophils to the alveolar cavity [46]. IL-17 also activated airway NEU by increasing elastase and myeloperoxidase activities, and promoted exacerbation of asthma [46]. It has shown that IL-17 may play an indirect role in airway remodeling of asthma, the increased concentration of IL-17 in PBMCs and plasma always implied that the asthmatic symptoms prone to more severe [47, 48]

IL-9 can be produced by a variety of cells including Th2 cells, Th9 cells, EOS and NEU [16], and Th9 cells were the main source of IL-9. Th9 cells promoted mast cell accumulation and activation in mice model of allergic pulmonary inflammation [49], while IL-9 can inhibit the production of IFN-γ and promote secretion of mucus and IgE [50, 51]. A study have found that both Th9 cell and IL-9 of peripheral blood increased in allergic asthma patients [52], which means that IL-9 can be regarded as a biomarker of asthma.

IL-25, IL-33 and TSLP derived from airway epithelium and played an important role in the pathogenesis of asthma [53]. Among them, IL-25 not only targeted innate immune cells to produce Th2 cytokines, but also guided the translation of naive Th cells to Th2 cells [54]. Overexpression of IL-25 in lung epithelium induced epithelial cell proliferation, increased mucus secretion, airway infiltration of eosinophils and macrophages, and up-regulated the chemokines related to Th2 cells [55]. Plasma IL-25 levels were also associated with epithelial IL-25 expression and may be useful for predicting responses to asthma therapy [56].

Genome wide and candidate gene association studies have identified that common single nucleotide polymorphisms (SNPs) in IL-33 and IL-1 receptor like 1 (IL-1RL1) loci associated with asthma, especially pediatric asthma [57]. IL-33 activated a large number of immune cells and structural cells by binding to IL-33 receptor complex, which can promote occurrence and exacerbation of asthma [58]. The IL-33/ST2 (suppression of tumorigenicity 2) axis triggered the release of several proinflammatory mediators, such as chemokines and cytokines, and induced systemic T2 inflammation in vivo [59]. IL-33/ST2 pathway also contributed to allergen induced airway inflammation and hyperresponsiveness [60]. Compared with healthy individuals, the concentration of IL-33 in plasma was higher in asthma patients [61].

To some extent, AHR, mucus overproduction and airway remodeling, were considered to be drived by TSLP through its downstream proinflammatory effect [62]. Stimulation of basophils with TSLP can increase the percentage of IL-25 receptor (IL-17RB) and ST2, suggesting that TSLP can enhance the responsiveness of basophils to other alarmin cytokines [63]. The levels of plasma TSLP in asthma patients were higher than that in healthy controls, Airway submucosal EOS would be reduced by blocking TSLP in patients with moderate-to-severe uncontrolled asthma compared with placebo [64].

2.4 Chemokine markers

Eotaxin, as a ESO chemokine, can attract EOS to the site of allergic inflammation by stimulating CCR3. Eotaxin played a role in the early stage of Th2 lymphocyte recruitment [65], and the concentration of airway eotaxin was related to the sensitivity of asthmatic airway [66]. A study has demonstrated that there was a direct relationship between asthma diagnosis and eotaxin, and the levels of plasma eotaxin were negatively correlated with pulmonary function [66].

CCR2 was expressed in monocytes and T lymphocytes [67]. CCR2 mediated release of monocyte precursors leads to the increase of lung dendritic cells (DC) in allergic airway inflammation [68]. A study showed that monocytes may modulate the inflammatory response in asthma [69]. In a mouse asthma model, CCL2/CCR2-dependent recruitment of Th17 cells to the lung promoted airway inflammation [70]. In a monkey asthma model, Neutralization of CCR2 reduced bronchial hyperreactivity and weakened the accumulation of macrophages and eosinophils in BALF [71]. Therefore, the elevated CCR2 was a diagnostic biomarker for asthma.

CCR3 was mainly expressed on EOS, and can also be detected on basophils and T cells [67]. CCR3 showed sequence homology in many species, including humans, mice and guinea pigs. Its expression was limited to cells involved in allergic inflammation [72]. MicroRNA-30a-3p (miR-30a-3p)can inhibit CCR3 signaling pathway, reduce the secretion of sIgE against ovalbumin (OVA), eotaxin, IL-5 and IL-4 [73]. The expression of CCR3 on the surface of PBMCs was positively correlated with severity of asthma [74]. Inhibition of CCR3 blocks eosinophil recruitment into the blood, lungs and airways and prevents AHR in a mouse asthma model [75].

CCR5 was expressed in T lymphocytes and macrophages [67]. The increased CCR5 lead to EOS accumulation and airway remodeling in asthma patients [76]. Compared with healthy subjects, the expression of CCR5 in peripheral blood lymphocytes increased in asthma patients, and inhibition of CCR5 was a feasible method for blocking AHR [77, 78].

Thymus and activation-regulated chemokine (TARC) was produced by DC, endothelial cells, keratinocytes, bronchial epithelial cells and fibroblasts [79]. As chemokine related T2 inflammation, TARC contributed to the activation of EOS and MC driven by Th2 [80]. A series of studies concluded that the TARC concentration of asthma children increased in plasma [81], and after treatment of systemic corticosteroid (CS), the concentration decreased. In addition, the levels of TARC were negatively correlated with indicator of lung function such as peak expiratory flow rates in asthma patients [82].

Monocyte chemotactic protein-4 (MCP-4) was a potential chemical attractant not only for EOS, but also for monocytes, lymphocytes and basophils [83]. It have been confirmed that MCP-4 can induce histamine release and activation of the EOS [74]. Plasma MCP-4 was higher in patients with acute asthma than in those with chronic stable asthma [83], which implied that MCP-4 was correlated with exacerbation of asthma.

2.5 Protein biomarkers

Heat shock protein 72 (HSP-72) belongs to the Hsp70 family of heat shock proteins. It regulated protein expression during conditions of cell stress and acted as a protective factor by preventing abnormal protein aggregation, thus helping to refold damaged proteins, which was related to inflammation and obesity. Obesity was considered to be a risk factor for asthma, and serum and urine Hsp72 levels were significantly elevated in patients with severe asthma and obesity-related asthma. Hsp72 also was an independent predictor of asthma severity and could be used as a simple, non-invasive biomarker for predicting and monitoring asthma severity in obese asthma patients [84].

Eosinophil cationic protein (ECP) was secreted by activated eosinophil and is a specific marker of EOS. Serum ECP levels were significantly increased in children and adults with allergic asthma during acute stage. ECP, as a strong alkali-toxic protein, had strong effects on airway and nasal epithelium and had been associated with AHR, eosinophilic chronic sinusitis, aspirin-aggravated respiratory disease, and recurrent wheezing [85]. Elevated ECP concentrations in serum reflected EOS activation and were associated with asthma severity and allergen sensitization. In children with acute asthma, serum ECP was a more sensitive biomarker of asthma severity than blood EOS [86].

Periostein was a matrix protein that expressed in fibroblasts and epithelial cells, which was involved in a variety of biological processes, such as cell proliferation, cell invasion, and angiogenesis. In asthma patients, periostein associated with EOS migration and promoted production Th2 cytokines such as IL-4 and IL-13, lead to chronic allergic inflammation. It was found that the best cut-off value of sputum periostein which distinguished mild and moderate to severe asthma was 528.25 ng/mL [87]. Serum periostein was associated with AHR, blood EOS counts and FeNO in asthma children. The level of sputum periosteins was positively correlated with age, asthma course and sputum EOS increase, which was a surrogate biomarker and therapeutic target of severe eosinophil asthma.

High mobility group protein B1 (HMGB1) was a protein that specifically binds to nucleosome DNA junction region, it can enhance nucleosome stability and transcription factor interaction. In asthma, acute respiratory distress syndrome (ARDS), cystic fibrosis, lung cancer and other lung diseases, HMGB1 induced the production of pro-inflammatory cytokines and exacerbated airway inflammation, and anti-HMGB1 can reduce the pathological features of asthma [88].

Serum chitinase-like protein YKL-40, a member of the chitinase family, might be involved in the development of fibrosis and airway remodeling. YKL-40 was involved in the pathogenesis of asthma by inducing IL-8 in the epithelium and was considered as one of the biomarkers of asthma patients [89]. In addition, YKL-40 also indicated neutrophil inflammation in asthma and was associated with asthma severity. Moreover, YKL-40 was significantly negatively correlated with lung function [90].

CD14 was a marker of activation of monocytes or macrophages, which existed in membrane-bound form (mCD14) and soluble form (sCD14) and had a positive effect on the balance between Th1 and Th2 cytokines. Soluble CD14(sCD14) played an important role in proliferation and activation of T and B cell. The level of sCD14 in asthma patients was significantly higher in the acute stage than in the convalescence stage. There was a significant correlation between plasma sCD14 level and the severity of asthma, lung function, asthma symptoms and signs in adults, and there was a negative correlation between sCD14 level and asthma severity [91]. Therefore, plasma sCD14 levels may be a potential biomarker for predicting asthma severity in adults.

Serum arginase I levels were significantly elevated in asthmatic patients compared with healthy controls and C-reactive protein (CRP) was a common inflammatory marker for assessing systemic inflammation. In asthma patients, serum high sensitivity CRP (HS-CRP) levels were elevated and associated with respiratory symptoms and airway inflammation. Serum arginase I level was positively correlated with HS-CRP and negatively correlated with IgE in asthma patients. Elevated serum arginase I levels might be serve as a biomarker of airway inflammation in asthma [92].

The OX40 ligand (OX40L,) and its receptor OX40 were members of the tumor necrosis factor (TNF) receptor superfamily. Serum OX40L was positively correlated with serum IgE, IL-6, percentage of EOS and NEU, TSLP, and negatively correlated with asthma severity and lung function. Inhaled corticosteroid (ICS) treatment can reduce serum OX40L levels, and the reduction of serum OX40L was more significant in steroid-sensitive asthma than in steroid-resistant asthma. High serum OX40L can be used as a biomarker for identifying glucocorticoid resistance in asthmatic patients. Changes in OX40L levels also reflect response to ICS treatment [93].

2.6 Non-coding RNA biomarkers

MicroRNAs (miRNAs) were small non-coding RNA molecules that were considered to be one of the basic regulatory mechanisms of gene expression. They were involved in many biological processes, such as signal transduction, cell proliferation and differentiation, apoptosis and stress response [94]. Sufficient evidence have been suggested that miRNA play a role in several key points of asthma, including the diagnosis of asthma, disease severity, and response to treatment [95].

Serum miRNA-21 and miRNA-155 levels were significantly elevated in asthma patients compared with healthy controls. The expression level of miRNA21 in serum of asthma patients was significantly positively correlated with the level of IL-4. In addition, compared with steroid-sensitive children, miRNA-21 was significantly elevated in untreated and steroid-resistant children, and miRNA-21 could be a promising biomarker for diagnosis and response to inhaled corticosteroid therapy [96].

MiR-20a-5p was significantly down-regulated in the lungs and OVA-stimulated cells of mouse models of OVA induced asthma, and miR-20a-5p may be a promising biomarker and therapeutic target during asthma progression by targeting ATG7's involvement in autophagy-induced apoptosis, fibrosis and inflammation [97]. MiR-582-5p was strongly upregulated in nasal epithelial cells of children with severe acute asthma [98]. MiR-145-5p was associated with lung function in children with asthma and also increased proliferation of airway smooth muscle cell. This suggests that the decreased expression of miR-145-5p was a risk factor for early decline in long-term lung function [99]. MiR-124 contributed to the development and maintenance of anti-inflammatory phenotypes of asthmatic lung macrophages, and was negatively correlated with the risk of exacerbation, severity and inflammation in asthma patients [100].

MiRNA-155, a key regulator of type 2 innate lymphocytes in a mouse model of allergic airway inflammation, was elevated in serum samples from allergic asthma patients compared with non-allergic asthma patients and healthy individuals. Expression of miR-155 was altered by allergic stimulation or glucocorticoid treatment, which can be used as biomarkers for steroids resistance/neutrophilic asthma [101]. MiRNA-223 was significantly upregulated in patients with moderate asthma compared with healthy controls, and no significant difference in miR-223 expression was found between patients with severe asthma and healthy controls, which could serve as a potential biomarker for the diagnosis of moderate asthma [102]. The level of miR-192 in asthma children was lower than that in healthy children, and miR-192 blocked the activation pathway of Tfh cells by targeting CXCR5 [103]. Serum miRNA-1165-3P levels were significantly elevated in asthma patients compared to healthy controls. In addition, Serum miR-1165-3p levels were also significantly elevated in patients with allergic rhinitis (AR) or allergic bronchopulmonary aspergillosis (ABPA), suggesting that serum miR-1165-3p may be used as a non-invasive biomarker to help diagnose and characterize allergic asthma [104]. MiRNA-3934 levels in peripheral blood mononuclear cells of asthma patients were significantly decreased, and miRNA-3934 levels in PBMCs could distinguish asthma patients, especially severe asthma patients from control group. MiRNA-3934 levels in PBMCs of asthma patients were negatively correlated with serum IL-6, IL-8 and IL-33 levels, respectively, which might also be a potential diagnostic biomarker for asthma [105]. In addition, upregulation of MiR-1165-3p reduced AHR and airway inflammation by directly targeting IL-13. MiR-185-5p was involved in calcium signaling by targeting NFAT and CaMKII proteins in cardiomyocytes and may play a role in muscle cell hyperplasia, proliferation and cell contraction in asthma, suggesting that these candidate biomarkers play a role in the pathogenesis of asthma [106]. Overexpression of MiRNA-126 in acute asthma was associated with signs of immune imbalance and can predicted disease severity, suggesting that it can be used as a potential serologic marker for the diagnosis and evaluation of asthma [107].

Long non-coding RNA (lncRNAs) affected the regulation of immune response, airway inflammation and other pathological processes related to asthma. PTTG3P was highly expressed in peripheral blood of children with asthma and promoted the progression of childhood asthma by targeting miR-192-3p/CCNB1 axis and may serve as a potential diagnostic and therapeutic biomarker for childhood asthma [108]. LncRNA NEAT1 was up-regulated in patients with asthma exacerbation compared with healthy controls and patients with asthma in remission stage, which was positively correlated with the severity of asthma exacerbation, TNF-α, IL-1β and IL-17, but negatively correlated with predicted IL-10, FEV1/FVC and FEV1%. Circulating lncRNA NEAT1 may be a novel biomarker for increased risk and severity of asthma exacerbations [100]. LncRNA-ANRIL/MiR-125a axis was upregulated in patients with acute asthma compared with those in remission and healthy subjects, and the LncRNA ANRIL/MiR-125a axis had good predictive value for the risk of bronchial asthma disease progression [109]. Compared with non-severe asthma patients, the expression of lncRNA GAS5 in PBMCs of severe asthma patients was increased. After treatment with CS in vitro, the expression of GAS5 was down-regulated in severe asthma patients, while up-regulated in non-severe asthma patients, highlighting the potential role of GAS5 as a biomarker for the diagnosis of severe asthma patients [110]. Compared with the healthy control group, the level of lncRNA-MEG3 in CD4+T cells of asthma patients was significantly increased, and the degree of Treg/Th17 imbalance was correlated with the severity of asthma mice symptoms. LncRNA-MEG3 can be used as a competitive endogenous RNA to inhibit the level of miRNA-17, miRNA-17 inhibits Th17 expression by directly targeting nuclear orphan receptor γ

T (RORγ T). Thus affecting Treg/Th17 balance in asthma, monitoring lncrNA-MEG3 in asthma patients can be used to judge the course of disease or recovery of patients [111]. The level of lnc-BAZ2B in children with allergic asthma was significantly higher than that in healthy children. Lnc-BAZ2B can aggravate allergen-induced pulmonary allergic inflammation by promoting the activation of M2 macrophages, which is positively correlated with the severity of asthma and blood eosinophil count. Thus, Lnc-BAZ2B plays a key role in exacerbating the progression of allergic asthma and may serve as a potential diagnostic marker for childhood asthma [112].

3. Conclusion

In conclusion, biomarkers were indicators of normal physiological processes, disease progression and response to treatment. Although many biomarkers for asthma have been mentioned in recent studies for the diagnosis of asthma, the identification of different phenotypes and efficacy evaluation, none of them have been approved for clinical practice so far, mainly due to their limited sensitivity and specificity. With the development of biomedicine, asthma research is moving from clinical symptoms, clinical phenotypes, lung function and medication response to genomics, proteomics, epigenetics, etc. More key molecules and biomarkers will be discovered in the future. Combined detection of multiple markers can more comprehensively analyze the patient's condition, thus providing more valuable clinical information for the diagnosis, classification and treatment of asthma, and ultimately achieving accurate diagnosis and treatment of asthma patients.

Author details

Chen Hao[1], Cui Yubao[2] and Zhu Rongfei[1*]

1 Department of Allergy, Tongji Hospital, Tongji Medical College, Huazhong University of Science and Technology, Wuhan, China

2 Clinical Research Center, The Affiliated Wuxi Hospital of Nanjing Medical University, Wuxi, China

*Address all correspondence to: zrf13092@163.com

IntechOpen

© 2022 The Author(s). Licensee IntechOpen. This chapter is distributed under the terms of the Creative Commons Attribution License (http://creativecommons.org/licenses/by/3.0), which permits unrestricted use, distribution, and reproduction in any medium, provided the original work is properly cited.

References

[1] Cloutier MM, Dixon AE, Krishnan JA, Lemanske RJ, Pace W, Schatz M. Managing Asthma in Adolescents and Adults: 2020 Asthma Guideline Update From the National Asthma Education and Prevention Program. JAMA. 2020;**324**:2301-2317

[2] Huang K, Yang T, Xu J, Yang L, Zhao J, Zhang X, et al. Prevalence, risk factors, and management of asthma in China: A national cross-sectional study. Lancet. 2019;**394**:407-418

[3] Lishen S, Qianlan Z, Yunxiao S. The Mechanism, testing, specific immunotherapy and anti-IgE therapy for allergic respiratory diseases in children. International Journal of Pediatrics. 2020;**47**:823-827

[4] Mendes FC, Paciencia I, Ferreira AC, Martins C, Rufo JC, Silva D, et al. Development and validation of exhaled breath condensate microRNAs to identify and endotype asthma in children. PLoS One. 2019;**14**:e224983

[5] Agache I, Akdis CA. Precision medicine and phenotypes, endotypes, genotypes, regiotypes, and theratypes of allergic diseases. The Journal of Clinical Investigation. 2019;**129**:1493-1503

[6] Pavord ID, Bel EH, Bourdin A, Chan R, Han JK, Keene ON, et al. From DREAM to REALITI-A and beyond: Mepolizumab for the treatment of eosinophil-driven diseases. Allergy. 2022;**77**:778-797

[7] Backman K, Nuolivirta K, Ollikainen H, Korppi M, Piippo-Savolainen E. Low eosinophils during bronchiolitis in infancy are associated with lower risk of adulthood asthma. Pediatric Allergy and Immunology. 2015;**26**:668-673

[8] Piippo-Savolainen E, Remes S, Korppi M. Does blood eosinophilia in wheezing infants predict later asthma? A prospective 18-20-year follow-up. Allergy and Asthma Proceedings. 2007;**28**:163-169

[9] Nadif R, Siroux V, Boudier A, le Moual N, Just J, Gormand F, et al. Blood granulocyte patterns as predictors of asthma phenotypes in adults from the EGEA study. The European Respiratory Journal. 2016;**48**:1040-1051

[10] Shamji MH, Layhadi JA, Scadding GW, Cheung D, Calderon MA, Turka LA, et al. Basophil expression of diamine oxidase: A novel biomarker of allergen immunotherapy response. The Journal of Allergy and Clinical Immunology. 2015;**135**:913-921

[11] Shamji MH, Kappen JH, Akdis M, Jensen-Jarolim E, Knol EF, Kleine-Tebbe J, et al. Biomarkers for monitoring clinical efficacy of allergen immunotherapy for allergic rhinoconjunctivitis and allergic asthma: An EAACI Position Paper. Allergy. 2017;**72**:1156-1173

[12] Brightling CE, Bradding P, Symon FA, Holgate ST, Wardlaw AJ, Pavord ID. Mast-cell infiltration of airway smooth muscle in asthma. The New England Journal of Medicine. 2002;**346**:1699-1705

[13] Bartemes KR, Kephart GM, Fox SJ, Kita H. Enhanced innate type 2 immune response in peripheral blood from patients with asthma. The Journal of Allergy and Clinical Immunology. 2014;**134**:671-678

[14] Smith SG, Chen R, Kjarsgaard M, Huang C, Oliveria JP, O'Byrne PM, et al. Increased numbers of activated group 2 innate lymphoid cells in the airways of patients with severe asthma and persistent airway eosinophilia. The Journal of Allergy and Clinical Immunology. 2016;**137**:75-86

[15] Sze E, Bhalla A, Nair P. Mechanisms and therapeutic strategies for non-T2 asthma. Allergy. 2020;**75**:311-325

[16] Hammad H, Lambrecht BN. The basic immunology of asthma. Cell. 2021;**184**:2521-2522

[17] Jeong J, Lee HK. The role of CD4(+) T cells and microbiota in the pathogenesis of asthma. International Journal of Molecular Sciences. 2021;**22**:11822

[18] Josefowicz SZ, Lu LF, Rudensky AY. Regulatory T cells: Mechanisms of differentiation and function. Annual Review of Immunology. 2012;**30**:531-564

[19] Mamessier E, Nieves A, Lorec AM, Dupuy P, Pinot D, Pinet C, et al. T-cell activation during exacerbations: A longitudinal study in refractory asthma. Allergy. 2008;**63**:1202-1210

[20] Saradna A, Do DC, Kumar S, Fu QL, Gao P. Macrophage polarization and allergic asthma. Translational Research. 2018;**191**:1-14

[21] Fitzpatrick AM, Holguin F, Teague WG, Brown LA. Alveolar macrophage phagocytosis is impaired in children with poorly controlled asthma. Journal of Allergy and Clinical Immunology. 2008;**121**:1378

[22] Gloudemans AK, Lambrecht BN, Smits HH. Potential of immunoglobulin A to prevent allergic asthma. Clinical & Developmental Immunology. 2013;**2013**:542091

[23] Ludviksson BR, Eiriksson TH, Ardal B, Sigfusson A, Valdimarsson H. Correlation between serum immunoglobulin A concentrations and allergic manifestations in infants. The Journal of Pediatrics. 1992;**121**:23-27

[24] Balzar S, Strand M, Nakano T, Wenzel SE. Subtle immunodeficiency in severe asthma: IgA and IgG2 correlate with lung function and symptoms. International Archives of Allergy and Immunology. 2006;**140**:96-102

[25] Szefler SJ, Wenzel S, Brown R, Erzurum SC, Fahy JV, Hamilton RG, et al. Asthma outcomes: Biomarkers. The Journal of Allergy and Clinical Immunology. 2012;**129**:S9-S23

[26] Holt PG, Strickland D, Bosco A, Belgrave D, Hales B, Simpson A, et al. Distinguishing benign from pathologic TH2 immunity in atopic children. The Journal of Allergy and Clinical Immunology. 2016;**137**:379-387

[27] Gandhi NA, Bennett BL, Graham NM, Pirozzi G, Stahl N, Yancopoulos GD. Targeting key proximal drivers of type 2 inflammation in disease. Nature Reviews. Drug Discovery. 2016;**15**:35-50

[28] Zhu J. T helper 2 (Th2) cell differentiation, type 2 innate lymphoid cell (ILC2) development and regulation of interleukin-4 (IL-4) and IL-13 production. Cytokine. 2015;**75**:14-24

[29] Swain SL, Weinberg AD, English M, Huston G. IL-4 directs the development of Th2-like helper effectors. Journal of Immunology. 1990;**145**:3796-3806

[30] Coyle AJ, Le Gros G, Bertrand C, Tsuyuki S, Heusser CH, Kopf M, et al. Interleukin-4 is required for the induction of lung Th2 mucosal immunity. American Journal of

Respiratory Cell and Molecular Biology. 1995;**13**:54-59

[31] Venkayya R, Lam M, Willkom M, Grunig G, Corry DB, Erle DJ. The Th2 lymphocyte products IL-4 and IL-13 rapidly induce airway hyperresponsiveness through direct effects on resident airway cells. American Journal of Respiratory Cell and Molecular Biology. 2002;**26**:202-208

[32] Stirling RG, van Rensen EL, Barnes PJ, Chung KF. Interleukin-5 induces CD34(+) eosinophil progenitor mobilization and eosinophil CCR3 expression in asthma. American Journal of Respiratory and Critical Care Medicine. 2001;**164**:1403-1409

[33] Shi H, Qin S, Huang G, Chen Y, Xiao C, Xu H, et al. Infiltration of eosinophils into the asthmatic airways caused by interleukin 5. American Journal of Respiratory Cell and Molecular Biology. 1997;**16**:220-224

[34] Robinson DS, Hamid Q, Ying S, Tsicopoulos A, Barkans J, Bentley AM, et al. Predominant TH2-like bronchoalveolar T-lymphocyte population in atopic asthma. The New England Journal of Medicine. 1992;**326**:298-304

[35] Ohnishi T, Kita H, Weiler D, Sur S, Sedgwick JB, Calhoun WJ, et al. IL-5 is the predominant eosinophil-active cytokine in the antigen-induced pulmonary late-phase reaction. The American Review of Respiratory Disease. 1993;**147**:901-907

[36] Punnonen J, Aversa G, Cocks BG, McKenzie AN, Menon S, Zurawski G, et al. Interleukin 13 induces interleukin 4-independent IgG4 and IgE synthesis and CD23 expression by human B cells. Proceedings of the National Academy of Sciences of the United States of America. 1993;**90**:3730-3734

[37] Hunninghake GM, Soto-Quiros ME, Avila L, Su J, Murphy A, Demeo DL, et al. Polymorphisms in IL13, total IgE, eosinophilia, and asthma exacerbations in childhood. The Journal of Allergy and Clinical Immunology. 2007;**120**:84-90

[38] Corren J. Role of interleukin-13 in asthma. Current Allergy and Asthma Reports. 2013;**13**:415-420

[39] Lee YC, Lee KH, Lee HB, Rhee YK. Serum levels of interleukins (IL)-4, IL-5, IL-13, and interferon-gamma in acute asthma. The Journal of Asthma. 2001;**38**:665-671

[40] Castro M, Corren J, Pavord ID, Maspero J, Wenzel S, Rabe KF, et al. Dupilumab efficacy and safety in moderate-to-severe uncontrolled asthma. The New England Journal of Medicine. 2018;**378**:2486-2496

[41] Eger K, Kroes JA, Ten BA, Bel EH. Long-term therapy response to Anti-IL-5 biologics in severe asthma: A real-life evaluation. The Journal of Allergy and Clinical Immunology. In Practice. 2021;**9**:1194-1200

[42] Bilsborough J, Leung DY, Maurer M, Howell M, Boguniewicz M, Yao L, et al. IL-31 is associated with cutaneous lymphocyte antigen-positive skin homing T cells in patients with atopic dermatitis. The Journal of Allergy and Clinical Immunology. 2006;**117**:418-425

[43] Yu JI, Han WC, Yun KJ, Moon HB, Oh GJ, Chae SC. Identifying polymorphisms in IL-31 and their association with susceptibility to asthma. Korean Journal of Pathology. 2012;**46**:162-168

[44] Datsi A, Steinhoff M, Ahmad F, Alam M, Buddenkotte J. Interleukin-31: The "itchy" cytokine in inflammation and therapy. Allergy. 2021;**76**:2982-2997

[45] Lai T, Wu D, Li W, Chen M, Yi Z, Huang D, et al. Interleukin-31 expression and relation to disease severity in human asthma. Scientific Reports. 2016;**6**:22835

[46] Ramakrishnan RK, Al HS, Hamid Q. Role of IL-17 in asthma pathogenesis and its implications for the clinic. Expert Review of Respiratory Medicine. 2019;**13**:1057-1068

[47] Molet S, Hamid Q, Davoine F, Nutku E, Taha R, Page N, et al. IL-17 is increased in asthmatic airways and induces human bronchial fibroblasts to produce cytokines. The Journal of Allergy and Clinical Immunology. 2001;**108**:430-438

[48] Zhao Y, Yang J, Gao YD, Guo W. Th17 immunity in patients with allergic asthma. International Archives of Allergy and Immunology. 2010;**151**:297-307

[49] Sehra S, Yao W, Nguyen ET, Glosson-Byers NL, Akhtar N, Zhou B, et al. TH9 cells are required for tissue mast cell accumulation during allergic inflammation. The Journal of Allergy and Clinical Immunology. 2015;**136**:433-440

[50] Jia L, Wang Y, Li J, Li S, Zhang Y, Shen J, et al. Detection of IL-9 producing T cells in the PBMCs of allergic asthmatic patients. BMC Immunology. 2017;**18**:38

[51] Louahed J, Toda M, Jen J, Hamid Q, Renauld JC, Levitt RC, et al. Interleukin-9 upregulates mucus expression in the airways. American Journal of Respiratory Cell and Molecular Biology. 2000;**22**:649-656

[52] Hoppenot D, Malakauskas K, Lavinskiene S, Bajoriuniene I, Kalinauskaite V, Sakalauskas R. Peripheral blood Th9 cells and eosinophil apoptosis in asthma patients. Medicina (Kaunas, Lithuania). 2015;**51**:10-17

[53] Mitchell PD, O'Byrne PM. Epithelial-derived cytokines in asthma. Chest. 2017;**151**:1338-1344

[54] Wang YH, Angkasekwinai P, Lu N, Voo KS, Arima K, Hanabuchi S, et al. IL-25 augments type 2 immune responses by enhancing the expansion and functions of TSLP-DC-activated Th2 memory cells. The Journal of Experimental Medicine. 2007;**204**:1837-1847

[55] Angkasekwinai P, Park H, Wang YH, Wang YH, Chang SH, Corry DB, et al. Interleukin 25 promotes the initiation of proallergic type 2 responses. The Journal of Experimental Medicine. 2007;**204**:1509-1517

[56] Cheng D, Xue Z, Yi L, Shi H, Zhang K, Huo X, et al. Epithelial interleukin-25 is a key mediator in Th2-high, corticosteroid-responsive asthma. American Journal of Respiratory and Critical Care Medicine. 2014;**190**:639-648

[57] El-Husseini ZW, Gosens R, Dekker F, Koppelman GH. The genetics of asthma and the promise of genomics-guided drug target discovery. The Lancet Respiratory Medicine. 2020;**8**:1045-1056

[58] Saikumar JA, Hesse L, Ketelaar ME, Koppelman GH, Nawijn MC. The central role of IL-33/IL-1RL1 pathway in asthma: From pathogenesis to intervention. Pharmacology & Therapeutics. 2021;**225**:107847

[59] Schmitz J, Owyang A, Oldham E, Song Y, Murphy E, McClanahan TK, et al. IL-33, an interleukin-1-like cytokine that signals via the IL-1

receptor-related protein ST2 and induces T helper type 2-associated cytokines. Immunity. 2005;**23**:479-490

[60] Kearley J, Buckland KF, Mathie SA, Lloyd CM. Resolution of allergic inflammation and airway hyperreactivity is dependent upon disruption of the T1/ST2-IL-33 pathway. American Journal of Respiratory and Critical Care Medicine. 2009;**179**:772-781

[61] Bhowmik M, Majumdar S, Dasgupta A, Gupta BS, Saha S. Pilot-scale study of human plasma proteomics identifies ApoE and IL33 as markers in atopic asthma. Journal of Asthma Allergy. 2019;**12**:273-283

[62] West EE, Kashyap M, Leonard WJ. TSLP: A key regulator of asthma pathogenesis. Drug Discovery Today Diseases Mechanism. 2012;**9**:e83-e88

[63] Salter BM, Oliveria JP, Nusca G, Smith SG, Tworek D, Mitchell PD, et al. IL-25 and IL-33 induce Type 2 inflammation in basophils from subjects with allergic asthma. Respiratory Research. 2016;**17**:5

[64] Diver S, Khalfaoui L, Emson C, Wenzel SE, Menzies-Gow A, Wechsler ME, et al. Effect of tezepelumab on airway inflammatory cells, remodelling, and hyperresponsiveness in patients with moderate-to-severe uncontrolled asthma (CASCADE): A double-blind, randomised, placebo-controlled, phase 2 trial. The Lancet Respiratory Medicine. 2021;**9**:1299-1312

[65] Lloyd CM, Delaney T, Nguyen T, Tian J, Martinez-A C, Coyle AJ, et al. CC chemokine receptor (CCR)3/eotaxin is followed by CCR4/monocyte-derived chemokine in mediating pulmonary T helper lymphocyte type 2 recruitment after serial antigen challenge in vivo. The Journal of Experimental Medicine. 2000;**191**:265-274

[66] Nakamura H, Weiss ST, Israel E, Luster AD, Drazen JM, Lilly CM. Eotaxin and impaired lung function in asthma. American Journal of Respiratory and Critical Care Medicine. 1999;**160**:1952-1956

[67] Murdoch C, Finn A. Chemokine receptors and their role in inflammation and infectious diseases. Blood. 2000;**95**:3032-3043

[68] Robays LJ, Maes T, Lebecque S, Lira SA, Kuziel WA, Brusselle GG, et al. Chemokine receptor CCR2 but not CCR5 or CCR6 mediates the increase in pulmonary dendritic cells during allergic airway inflammation. Journal of Immunology. 2007;**178**:5305-5311

[69] Al-Rashoudi R, Moir G, Al-Hajjaj MS, Al-Alwan MM, Wilson HM, Crane IJ. Differential expression of CCR2 and CX3CR1 on CD16(+) monocyte subsets is associated with asthma severity. Allergy, Asthma and Clinical Immunology. 2019;**15**:64

[70] Wang A, Wang Z, Cao Y, Cheng S, Chen H, Bunjhoo H, et al. CCL2/CCR2-dependent recruitment of Th17 cells but not Tc17 cells to the lung in a murine asthma model. International Archives of Allergy and Immunology. 2015;**166**:52-62

[71] Mellado M, Martin DAA, Gomez L, Martinez C, Rodriguez-Frade JM. Chemokine receptor 2 blockade prevents asthma in a cynomolgus monkey model. The Journal of Pharmacology and Experimental Therapeutics. 2008;**324**:769-775

[72] Pease JE, Williams TJ. Eotaxin and asthma. Current Opinion in Pharmacology. 2001;**1**:248-253

[73] Li X, Wang B, Huang M, Wang X. miR-30a-3p participates in the development of asthma by targeting CCR3. Open Medicine. 2020;**15**:483-491

[74] Lun SW, Wong CK, Ko FW, Ip WK, Hui DS, Lam CW. Aberrant expression of CC and CXC chemokines and their receptors in patients with asthma. Journal of Clinical Immunology. 2006;**26**:145-152

[75] Grozdanovic M, Laffey KG, Abdelkarim H, Hitchinson B, Harijith A, Moon HG, et al. Novel peptide nanoparticle-biased antagonist of CCR3 blocks eosinophil recruitment and airway hyperresponsiveness. The Journal of Allergy and Clinical Immunology. 2019;**143**:669-680

[76] Schuh JM, Blease K, Hogaboam CM. The role of CC chemokine receptor 5 (CCR5) and RANTES/CCL5 during chronic fungal asthma in mice. The FASEB Journal. 2002;**16**:228-230

[77] Rojas-Dotor S, Segura-MendezNH,Miyagui-NamikawaK, Mondragon-Gonzalez R. Expression of resistin, CXCR3, IP-10, CCR5 and MIP-1alpha in obese patients with different severity of asthma. Biological Research. 2013;**46**:13-20

[78] Gauthier M, Kale SL, Oriss TB, Scholl K, Das S, Yuan H, et al. Dual role for CXCR3 and CCR5 in asthmatic type 1 inflammation. The Journal of Allergy and Clinical Immunology. 2022;**149**:113-124

[79] Saeki H, Tamaki K. Thymus and activation regulated chemokine (TARC)/CCL17 and skin diseases. Journal of Dermatological Science. 2006;**43**:75-84

[80] Luu QQ, Moon JY, Lee DH, Ban GY, Kim SH, Park HS. Role of thymus and activation-regulated chemokine in allergic asthma. Journal of Asthma Allergy. 2022;**15**:157-167

[81] Leung TF, Wong CK, Chan IH, Ip WK, Lam CW, Wong GW. Plasma concentration of thymus and activation-regulated chemokine is elevated in childhood asthma. The Journal of Allergy and Clinical Immunology. 2002;**110**:404-409

[82] Leung TF, Wong CK, Lam CW, Li AM, Ip WK, Wong GW, et al. Plasma TARC concentration may be a useful marker for asthmatic exacerbation in children. The European Respiratory Journal. 2003;**21**:616-620

[83] Kalayci O, Sonna LA, Woodruff PG, Camargo CJ, Luster AD, Lilly CM. Monocyte chemotactic protein-4 (MCP-4; CCL-13): A biomarker of asthma. The Journal of Asthma. 2004;**41**:27-33

[84] Soliman NA, Abdel GM, El KR, Hafez YM, Abo ER, Atef MM. Cross talk between Hsp72, HMGB1 and RAGE/ERK1/2 signaling in the pathogenesis of bronchial asthma in obese patients. Molecular Biology Reports. 2020;**47**:4109-4116

[85] Jiang XG, Yang XD, Lv Z, Zhuang PH. Elevated serum levels of TNF-alpha, IL-8, and ECP can be involved in the development and progression of bronchial asthma. The Journal of Asthma. 2018;**55**:111-118

[86] Rydell N, Nagao M, Moverare R, Ekoff H, Sjolander A, Borres MP, et al. Serum eosinophilic cationic protein is a reliable biomarker for childhood asthma. International Archives of Allergy and Immunology. 2022;**183**:744-752

[87] Refaat MM, El SE, Abd EW, Elbanna AH, Sayed H. Relationship between sputum periostin level and

inflammatory asthma phenotypes in Egyptian patients. The Journal of Asthma. 2021;**58**:1285-1291

[88] Hwang YH, Lee Y, Paik MJ, Yee ST. Inhibitions of HMGB1 and TLR4 alleviate DINP-induced asthma in mice. Toxicological Research (Camb). 2019;**8**:621-629

[89] Baos S, Calzada D, Cremades L, Sastre J, Quiralte J, Florido F, et al. Biomarkers associated with disease severity in allergic and nonallergic asthma. Molecular Immunology. 2017;**82**:34-45

[90] Yildiz H, Alp HH, Sunnetcioglu A, Ekin S, Mermit CB. Evaluation serum levels of YKL-40, Periostin, and some inflammatory cytokines together with IL-37, a new anti-inflammatory cytokine, in patients with stable and exacerbated asthma. Heart & Lung. 2021;**50**:177-183

[91] Zhou T, Huang X, Ma J, Zhou Y, Liu Y, Xiao L, et al. Association of plasma soluble CD14 level with asthma severity in adults: A case control study in China. Respiratory Research. 2019;**20**:19

[92] Ogino K, Obase Y, Takahashi N, Shimizu H, Takigawa T, Wang DH, et al. High serum arginase I levels in asthma: Its correlation with high-sensitivity C-reactive protein. The Journal of Asthma. 2011;**48**:1-7

[93] Ma SL, Zhang L. Elevated serum OX40L is a biomarker for identifying corticosteroid resistance in pediatric asthmatic patients. BMC Pulmonary Medicine. 2019;**19**:66

[94] Specjalski K, Niedoszytko M. MicroRNAs: Future biomarkers and targets of therapy in asthma? Current Opinion in Pulmonary Medicine. 2020;**26**:285-292

[95] Rial MJ, Canas JA, Rodrigo-Munoz JM, Valverde-Monge M, Sastre B, Sastre J, et al. Changes in serum MicroRNAs after Anti-IL-5 biological treatment of severe asthma. International Journal of Molecular Sciences. 2021;**22**:1-9

[96] ElKashef S, Ahmad SE, Soliman Y, Mostafa MS. Role of microRNA-21 and microRNA-155 as biomarkers for bronchial asthma. Innate Immunity. 2021;**27**:61-69

[97] Yu Y, Men S, Zhang Y. miR-20a-5p ameliorates ovalbumin (OVA)-induced mouse model of allergic asthma through targeting ATG7-regulated cell death, fibrosis and inflammation. International Immunopharmacology. 2021;**95**:107342

[98] Trifunovic A, Dombkowski A, Cukovic D, Mahajan P. The potential of microRNAs as noninvasive biomarkers in acute pediatric asthma. The Journal of Allergy and Clinical Immunology. 2020;**145**:1706-1708

[99] Tiwari A, Li J, Kho AT, Sun M, Lu Q, Weiss ST, et al. COPD-associated miR-145-5p is downregulated in early-decline FEV1 trajectories in childhood asthma. The Journal of Allergy and Clinical Immunology. 2021;**147**:2181-2190

[100] Li X, Ye S, Lu Y. Long non-coding RNA NEAT1 overexpression associates with increased exacerbation risk, severity, and inflammation, as well as decreased lung function through the interaction with microRNA-124 in asthma. Journal of Clinical Laboratory Analysis. 2020;**34**:e23023

[101] Weidner J, Ekerljung L, Malmhall C, Miron N, Radinger M. Circulating microRNAs correlate to clinical parameters in individuals with allergic and non-allergic asthma. Respiratory Research. 2020;**21**:107

[102] Rostami HS, Alizadeh Z, Mazinani M, Mahlooji RM, Fazlollahi MR, Kazemnejad A, et al. Exosomal MicroRNAs as Biomarkers in Allergic Asthma. Iranian Journal of Allergy, Asthma, and Immunology. 2021;**20**:160-168

[103] Zhang D, Wu Y, Sun G. miR-192 suppresses T follicular helper cell differentiation by targeting CXCR5 in childhood asthma. Scandinavian Journal of Clinical and Laboratory Investigation. 2018;**78**:236-242

[104] Wu C, Xu K, Wang Z, Chen Z, Sun Z, Yu W, et al. A novel microRNA miR-1165-3p as a potential diagnostic biomarker for allergic asthma. Biomarkers. 2019;**24**:56-63

[105] Wang W, Wang J, Chen H, Zhang X, Han K. Downregulation of miR-3934 in peripheral blood mononuclear cells of asthmatic patients and its potential diagnostic value. BioMed Research International. 2021;**2021**:8888280

[106] Xu L, Yi M, Tan Y, Yi Z, Zhang Y. A comprehensive analysis of microRNAs as diagnostic biomarkers for asthma. Therapeutic Advances in Respiratory Disease. 2020;**14**:1022250393

[107] Tian M, Ji Y, Wang T, Zhang W, Zhou Y, Cui Y. Changes in circulating microRNA-126 levels are associated with immune imbalance in children with acute asthma. International Journal of Immunopathology and Pharmacology. 2018;**32**:1680016491

[108] Dai B, Sun F, Cai X, Li C, Liu F, Shang Y. Long noncoding RNA PTTG3P/miR-192-3p/CCNB1 axis is a potential biomarker of childhood asthma. International Immunopharmacology. 2021;**101**:108229

[109] Ye S, Zhu S, Feng L. LncRNA ANRIL/miR-125a axis exhibits potential as a biomarker for disease exacerbation, severity, and inflammation in bronchial asthma. Journal of Clinical Laboratory Analysis. 2020;**34**:e23092

[110] Wu D, Gu B, Qian Y, Sun Y, Chen Y, Mao ZD, et al. Long non-coding RNA growth arrest specific-5: A potential biomarker for early diagnosis of severe asthma. Journal of Thoracic Disease. 2020;**12**:1960-1971

[111] Qiu YY, Wu Y, Lin MJ, Bian T, Xiao YL, Qin C. LncRNA-MEG3 functions as a competing endogenous RNA to regulate Treg/Th17 balance in patients with asthma by targeting microRNA-17/ RORgammat. Biomedicine & Pharmacotherapy. 2019;**111**:386-394

[112] Xia L, Wang X, Liu L, Fu J, Xiao W, Liang Q, et al. lnc-BAZ2B promotes M2 macrophage activation and inflammation in children with asthma through stabilizing BAZ2B pre-mRNA. The Journal of Allergy and Clinical Immunology. 2021;**147**:921-932

Chapter 4

Environmental and Occupational Factors; Contribution and Perspectives on Difficult to Treat Asthma

Christian Castillo Latorre, Sulimar Morales Colon, Alba D. Rivera Diaz, Vanessa Fonseca Ferrer, Mariana Mercader Perez, Ilean Lamboy Hernandez, Luis Gerena Montano, William Rodriguez Cintron and Onix Cantres Fonseca

Abstract

There are multiple well-recognized environmental factors that contribute to asthma exacerbation. Exposures to many of them will get unrecognized and most of the time will remain constant without knowing it is the causative agent. For an early identification of exposures and causative agents, a systematic approach needs to be taken in consideration by the encountering physician. Multiple questionnaires had been implementing and discussing organic and inorganic factors as well intrinsic and extrinsic factors. It is well-recognized that environmental exposures can cause worsening of asthma, other allergic conditions and even more severe pulmonary diseases. Asthma is a very prevalent disease with increased incidence nowadays. In the last decade, multiple new medications had been discovered for the treatment of moderate-to-severe persistent asthma, which most of them target the cellular component of the disease such as eosinophils and specific Immunoglobins. In the era of personalized medicine, environmental and occupational factors in asthma are key players that need to be recognized early in this patient population. In this chapter will go over model of effects, mechanism of action of these environmental factors, recognition, course of action and management of this patient population.

Keywords: environmental factors, occupational factors, exacerbation, allergens and irritants, asthma

1. Introduction

There are usually multiple risk factors that could exacerbate patients with asthma and other respiratory diseases. There are some risk factors that can be recognized

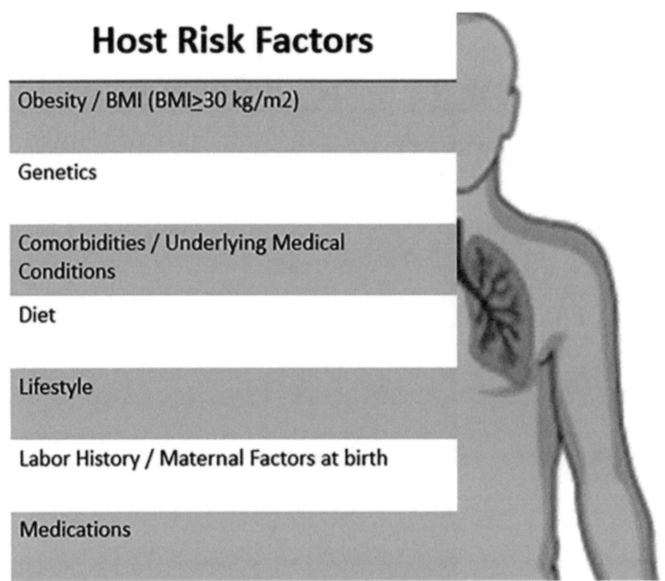

Figure 1.
Host factors contributing to asthma exacerbations.

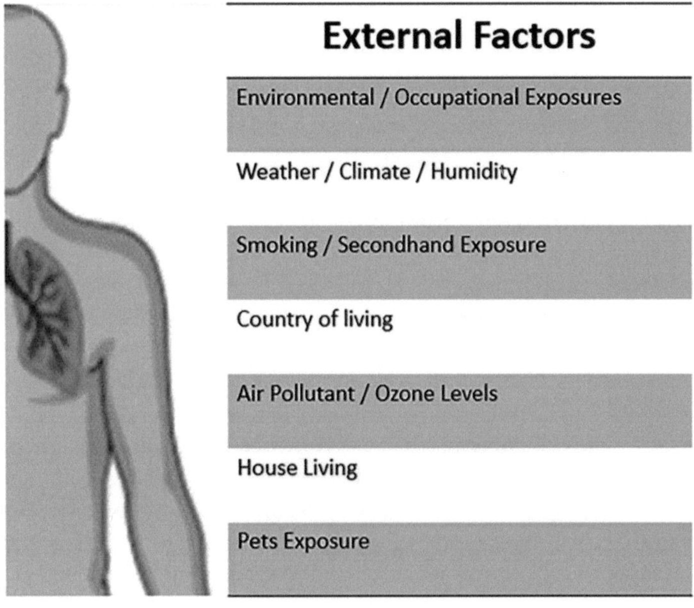

Figure 2.
External environmental and occupational factors.

quickly such as family history, smoking history and animals. There are Host factors contributing that contribute to asthma exacerbations (**Figure 1**), and external risk factors (**Figure 2**). further recognized other not so clear risk factors good understanding of asthma pathophysiology needs to be study. Asthma is a heterogeneous disease, characterized by airway hyperresponsiveness, chronic airway inflammation, reversible airway obstruction and remodeling of the lung, leading to respiratory symptoms, which includes shortness of breath, wheezes, chest tightness and cough [1]. These symptoms vary over time in intensity and are present with variable expiratory airflow limitation [2]. However, airflow limitation may become persistent later in the course of the disease, making this condition difficult to treat [3]. Diagnosing asthma in the setting of multiple environmental factors is a challenging work, however at some point patients will lead the physician for specific factors that worsens the disease. Irritant's exposures will lead to asthma symptoms in specific situations which makes this heterogenous disease sometimes a predictable one [4]. Uncontrolled asthma is when patient has either poor symptom control (frequent symptoms or increased use of rescue therapy, when have limited activity due to asthma, night waking due to asthma or have frequent exacerbation, defined as more than 2 exacerbations a year requiring oral corticosteroids or serious exacerbations (> 1/year) requiring hospitalization [3]. Difficult to treat asthma is when there is poor symptom control, despite patient been on optimal therapy. Optimal therapy includes maintenance treatment with medium or high dose inhaled corticosteroids (ICS) or oral corticosteroids with a second controller, which is usually a long-acting beta agonist (LABA) or with maintenance of oral corticosteroids.

It is known that asthma is a multifactorial condition that includes a combination of genetic and environmental factors [5]. Early recognition is critical in the proper management of asthma, as well as to prevent exacerbations and complications [6].

Environmental factors induce airway inflammation that leads to an exaggerated hypersensitivity that cause airway obstruction [5]. This response is the result of an increased presence of eosinophils, lymphocytes, and mast cells leading to airway inflammation and damage to the bronchial epithelium. The most common cause is IgE-mediated type I allergen exposure response [7]. Environmental factors that contribute to asthma symptoms and severity include viral infection, allergens (cockroaches, dust mites, pollens, animal dander and molds), indoor and outdoor air pollution, tobacco smoke (passive and active smoker), occupational sensitizers (isocyanates, platinum salts, animal biological products), and other causes such as exercise food allergies, GERD, Aspirin or NSAID sensitivity, among others. Occupational asthma is an important part of the environmental factors that contribute to difficult to treat asthma. Occupational exposures are a major cause of lung disease and disability worldwide [8, 9]. It is estimated that work related exposures account for as much as 15–25% of the asthma burden in the United States [10]. Work-related asthma may cause functional impairment and disability and tends to cause higher morbidity than general asthma [11]. In new cases of asthma presentation in adults with an unknown trigger, work-related asthma should be considered.

1.1 Work-related asthma (WRA)

Early recognition of this entity and control of exposures are important in work-related induced asthma, because low-molecular-weight chemical sensitizers, also cause asthma in a similar mechanism of allergens [7]. WRA is divided into 2 categories: (1) Occupational asthma (OA), which is define as the asthma that is caused by exposition of an agent at work and (2) Work exacerbated asthma (WEA), with is defined as pre-existing asthma that is exacerbated by exposure to an agent at work· OA is suggested by a correlation between asthma symptoms and work, as well as with improvement when away from work for several days. It is cause by agents that are classified depending on their molecular weight; high-molecular-weight (HMW) or low molecular weight (LMW) agents [12]. The HMW antigens consist of animal and plant proteins, fungi, and other large organic molecules. The LMW antigens consist of chemicals and some metal salts [13].

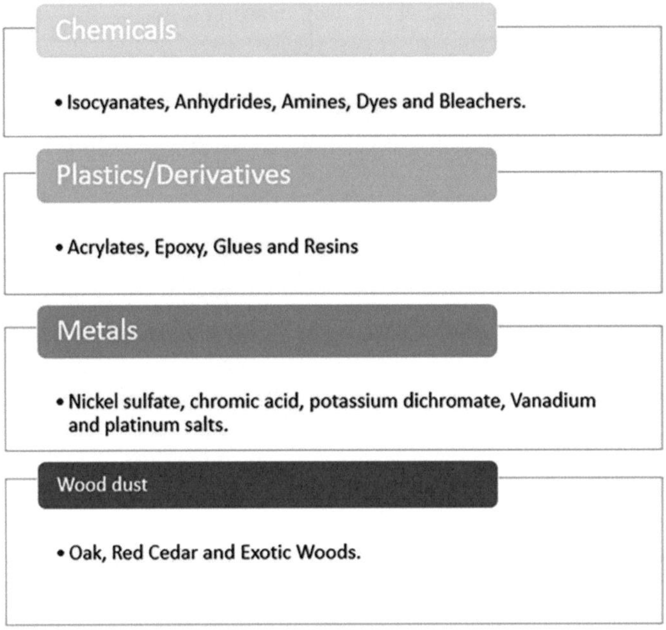

Chemicals

- Isocyanates, Anhydrides, Amines, Dyes and Bleachers.

Plastics/Derivatives

- Acrylates, Epoxy, Glues and Resins

Metals

- Nickel sulfate, chromic acid, potassium dichromate, Vanadium and platinum salts.

Wood dust

- Oak, Red Cedar and Exotic Woods.

Figure 3.
Inorganic occupational exposures contributing to difficult to treat asthma.

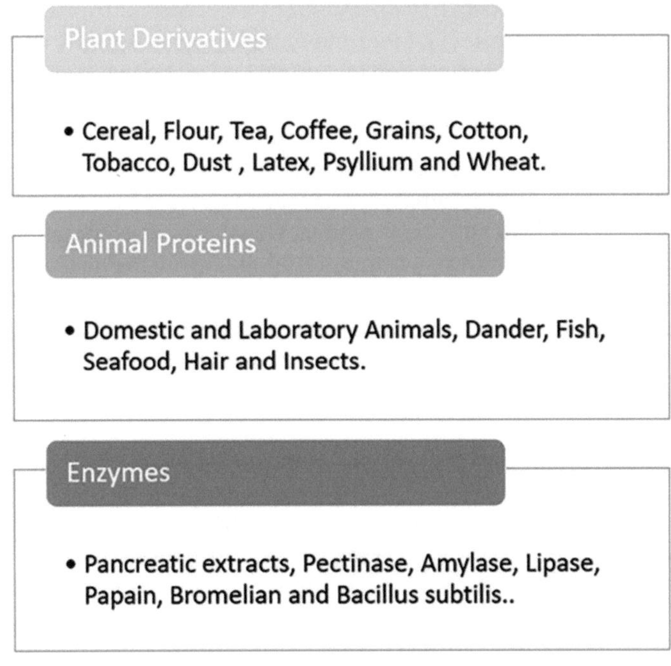

Figure 4.
Organic occupational exposures contributing to difficult to treat asthma.

It is thought that the LMW act through type I hypersensitivity mechanism, producing specific IgE antibodies, but the entire mechanisms are not well understood [12]. It is know that offending agents can cause an acute inflammatory response inducing reactive

Major Occupational Asthma Causes		
Offending agent	Examples	Occupation/Environment at risk
Low molecular weight irritant		
Drugs	• Beta-lactam antibiotics, opiates	Pharmaceutical workers, farm workers, health professionals
Chemical dust and vapors	• Isocyanates → Hexamethylene diisocyanate, toluene diisocyanate, diphenylmethane diisocyanate, naphthalene diisocyanate. • Anhydrides → Phthalic anhydride, trimellitic anhydride • Amines → Quaternary amines, chloramine. • Dyes and bleaches → Henna extract, anthraquinone, reactive dyes, carmine, persulfate.	Manufacturers of many industries such as upholstery, foam mattresses, insulation, polyurethane, plastics, paints and platers, welders, metal and chemical workers, packaging materials
Plastics and derivatives	• Acrylates, epoxy, other glues and resins	Plastic and resin manufacturers
Wood dust	• Oak, red cedar, exotic woods	Carpenters, woodworker
Metals	• Nickel sulfate, chromic acid, potassium dichromate, vanadium, platinum salts.	Welders, platers, metal and chemical workers
High molecular weight irritant		
Organic dust (Plant and Animal Substances)	• Plant derivatives → Cereals, flour, tea, coffee, grains, cotton, tobacco dust, latex, psyllium, wheat. • Animal Proteins → Domestic and laboratory animals, dander, fish, seafood, hair, small insects. • Enzymes → Pancreatic extracts, pectinase, amylase, lipase, papain, bromelain, *Bacillus subtilis*.	Farmers, cotton and textile workers, carpenters, woodworker, dusts from cotton and textile manufacture, veterinarians, dock workers, bakers, food processors, detergent manufacturers, health and pharmaceutical professionals, animal handlers

Figure 5.
*Major occupational asthma causes divided by molecular weight into low molecular weight irritant and high molecular weight irritant. **Rosenman KD, Beckett WS. Web based listing of agents associated with new onset work-related asthma. Respir med. 2015 may; 109(5):625–31.*

airways dysfunction syndrome, if exposure is repeated a chronic inflammation is produced that leads to persistent or permanent changes consistent with asthma [12]. It is important to recognize this offending agent as early as possible to prevent these changes. The most frequent causes of OA are Flour (31%) Isocyanates (17%), Persulfates (7%), Metals (4%), Wood (3%), Latex (3%), Acylates (3%), Quaternary ammonium (3.2%), Others (28%) [13], this factors can be divided into inorganic (**Figure 3**) and organic (**Figure 4**) risk factors, high molecular and low molecular weight (**Figure 5**).

**Torén K, Brisman J, Olin AC, Blanc PD. Asthma on the job: work-related factors in new onset-asthma and in exacerbations of pre-existing asthma. Respir Med. 2000 Jun;94(6):529–35.

2. Clinical assessment: physical examination and medical history

The signs and symptoms of asthma vary widely among every individual, as well as over time. This reversible airway obstruction pulmonary disease is characterized by the presence of several symptoms including nonproductive cough, chest tightness, episodic wheezing and dyspnea usually brought spontaneously or after exposures of identified triggers or stimuli and relieved or improved with the use of bronchodilator therapy. Diagnosis is often difficult, as clinical presentation is nonspecific and my overlap with other comorbidities. The diagnosis of asthma involves a careful and detailed process of history taking, physical examination, laboratory studies and diagnostic studies which demonstrate variable expiratory airflow obstruction [14]. Asthma can affect any age, but is more common during childhood years, till many patients may have a remission of the disease during puberty with recurrence of the disease once day enter adulthood. Most cases of adult-onset asthma are usually related to occupational exposure, associated with aspirin induced or described as an eosinophilic type of asthma [15]. When evaluating a patient with suspected asthma; history taking should focus on aspects such as the presence of symptoms, the pattern and frequency of such symptoms, what are some precipitating factors and the existence of atopy, among other risk factors. There are some physical examination findings (**Figure 6**), which increase the likelihood of asthma and include the presence of nasal secretions, nasal swelling, and presence of nasal polyps, which are common in patients with allergic asthma. Cough may be dry or productive, where sputum have a pale yellowish discoloration which is secondary to presence of eosinophils and usually worsen at night. Chest tightness is most like band like, with feeling of heavy chest compression. Atopic dermatitis and eczemas are the most common skin manifestation noted in patients with asthma.

Chest examination may be normal between exacerbation, but during exacerbations there is limited airflow to cause wheezing, for which patients present with reduced breath sounds with prolonged expiration. Tripod position, use of accessory muscle of respiration and prolonged expiration (defined as decreased I: E ratio), are also noted during acute asthma exacerbations.

There are several risk factors that are involved in the development of asthma and many of them are an interaction between both host and environmental factors. Several studies have identified genetic factors that predispose to asthma, but these interact with other environmental factors such as indoor allergens such as furred

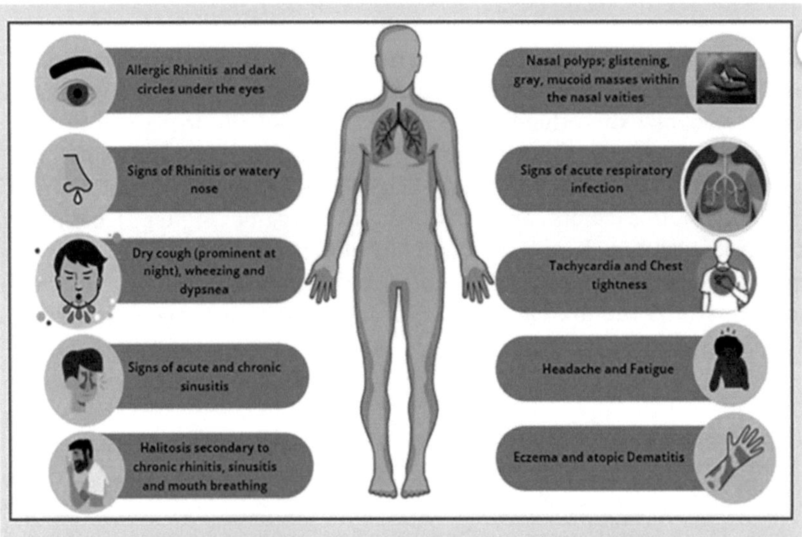

Figure 6.
Common clinical features in difficult to treat asthma that relates to environmental and occupational exposures.

animals, dusts, rodents, mold and cockroaches, as well as outdoor allergens as mols, pollen, air pollution, fumes, occupational exposure, and viral infections. History of tobacco smoking, second hand smoking exposure and commodities such as obesity, are also important risk factors. A personal history or family history of atopy may be present, characterized by seasonal allergies, atopic dermatitis and conjunctivitis, is common. There are cases, where patients have sensitivity to aspirin, presence of nasal polyps and wheezing, commonly known as the "asthmatic triad". This specific asthma symptoms, can be further recognized and attributed to specific situations were an environmental or occupation factors is present. When dealing with environmental exposures one of the most common symptoms that patients will be expressing is sneezing, rhinitis, and shortness of breath that can be divided in to dry cough or chest tightness, that most of the time will lead to increase in asthma regimens. Most of the patients will have some kind of relieve when they completely avoid this exposures such as vacation times or time off at home, however most of the environmental factors present at work place environmental can be found at home.

2.1 Diagnostic modalities

Establishing the diagnosis of asthma requires evaluation with a pulmonary function test (PFT). Other test such as laboratory testing, chest x-rays and allergy testing are mainly used to identify the different phenotypes of asthma. Arterial blood gas examination is also use and help to identify those patients with respiratory acidosis or increase CO_2 that are in impending respiratory failure and may require mechanical ventilation as part of their treatment. In severe exacerbation, patients may present with hypoxemia and increase alveolar to arterial oxygen gradient, requiring oxygen supplementation. The PFT determines the degree and reversibility of airflow obstruction. Spirometry prior and after bronchodilation therapy is used for proper evaluation of the forced expiratory volume in one second (FEV_1, forced vital capacity (FVC) and FEV_1/FVC ratio. These measurements aid in the determination of airflow obstruction and reversibility of the disease. Airflow obstruction is defined as a ratio of FEV_1 to FVC less than 0.70 or less than lower limit of normal. Severity of the disease is determined by the degree of reduction in the FEV_1 below normal values. Patient with a FEV_1 more than 70% predicted are classify as mild obstruction, a FEV_1 between 50 to 69% predicted have moderate obstruction and FEV_1 less than 50% predicted have severe obstruction [16]. Reversibility is determined by an increase of 12% or more than 200 ml in the FEV_1 or FVC after the use of inhaled bronchodilators. Diagnostic modalities such as peak flow meters can be used when specific environmental factors are present and it will lead to variability of flow at this situations, and disappearance of this reduction in flows when not at contact.

In patients where spirometry is not diagnostic, a bronchial provocation testing with methacholine or histamine is used to diagnose asthma. A positive testing is defined as a reduction in the FEV_1 of 20% or more or 8 mg/ml. When patient have a negative result there is 95% chance of ruling out asthma as the diagnosis, due to this testing high negative predictive value. Another important tool that is used to monitor or quantify asthma severity is the Peak Flow. This serves as an objective tool used by clinicians and patients, to monitor flow variability and response to medical treatment. Peak flow depends on patient's height, weight and age but these are poorly standardized markers and measurement tends to vary as the day goes by. It is recommended that peak flow be used early in the morning after the use of bronchodilator therapy and in the afternoon. Patients that have a change of 20% or more from morning measurements or from day to day, suggest that patients have an uncontrolled asthma and required medication adjustments. If there is less than 200 L/min then there is severe airflow obstruction [16].

Imaging studies are not routinely done, as most patient have normal chest X ray. Some patients may show hyperinflation, diminished peripheral vasculature and bronchial thickening. Chest imaging are usually done when other superimpose conditions are suspected such as pneumonia or pneumothorax are suspected. Skin testing in combination with serum IgE leves is sometimes used together to better evaluate patients with atopy and aeroallergens, which in some cases will provide clinically relevant information. Absolute eosinophil count is requested for evaluation of eosinophilic asthma which benefit from anti IlL5 monotherapy. Finally, evaluation of the paranasal sinus and esophagus is done to rule out gastroesophageal reflux disease or paranasal sinus disease as a possible cause for refractory or persistent asthma.

3. Environmental and occupational triggers of asthma

The purpose of this section is to review indoor air pollution factors that contribute to asthma exacerbation, not controlled symptoms and difficult to treat disease. Its important to note that we spend most of the time in the indoor environment which makes this environment the most susceptible to this patient population, and most of the time very difficult to control. When we are dealing with a difficult to treat asthma patient, we need to have a good sense of the patient surroundings such as work, home and most visited places during the day. Analysis of time exposure with symptoms is important, to down-regulate possibilities and get to the causative factor. The steps to establishing causative and effect relationship between exposures is a complicated and essential component in management patients with strong environmental effects. Discussion will be made separating indoor with outdoor environmental factors, as well most recognized causative agents.

3.1 Indoor air pollution

There are many sources of indoor air pollution, which can be increase with outdoor pollutions contaminant. Exposure to indoor air pollutants can cause detrimental health issues, which could cause minor symptoms such as allergies represented with constant sneezing, coughing which can be exacerbated with indoor change in temperatures and irritants [17]. This irritant could cause only upper respiratory symptoms; however, it could get complicated with lower respiratory symptoms such as reactive airway disease and bronchial asthma exacerbations in patients with underlying hyperactive airways. It's important to note that indoor environments will get outdoor mixtures of pollutants in which will reaccumulate with indoor sources causing a conjoined effect. Indoor factors could range from animal matters, molds from humid areas, secondhand tobacco exposure and dust mites among others that will be further discuss.

3.2 Particulate matter

It consists of particles suspended in the air which can be from human sources such as factories, vehicles, personal or community transports, electricity plants and industrial fumes, or natural matters such as pollen, spontaneous fires, spores, animal debris and plants among others. It's important to note that particulate matter can be divided with sizes going from particles less than 10 um in diameter (PM10) to particles less than 2.5 um (PM2.5) [18]. One of the strongest clinical differences between this particle is that particles less than 10 um could enter the respiratory system, and the smallest ones will be able to enter the alveoli which is the distal component of the airway. Particles that are between 2.5 um to 10 um will not be able to reach the alveoli but will be possible to deposit in the more proximal airways in which the clinical sequela will be different. With this it's important to point out that proximal airway deposition will have a clinical presentation of asthma, with reactive airway disease, which may cause inflammation and subsequent exacerbation of underlying asthma. Multiple studies have shown that strong particulate exposure led to lower pulmonary function and deterioration overtime [19]. Physiology of particulate matter starts when it enters the body through the nose and mouth when we are breathing, at that moment the body will be able to eliminate most of the largest particles which are the ones more than 2.5 um, but the other smaller particles will continue passage into the lungs and have detrimental stationary inflammatory effects in the alveoli. This effect could lead to interstitial lung disease with permanent parenchyma damage as well acute diseases such as hypersensitivity pneumonitis, chronic bronchitis among others [20]. It will not only lead to respiratory symptoms if can case cardiovascular complications such as arrhythmia and coronary artery disease. This makes particulate matter a detrimental environmental factor to the healthy people but most importantly to patients with comorbidities such as asthma.

3.3 Indoor nitrogen dioxide

Nitrogen dioxide is an irritant gas that has strongly been linked with respiratory symptoms with negative long term sequelas. It's a product of elevated temperature combustion as can been seen in indoor gasses such as indoor stoves. There are other sources of NO2 such as power plants which is specifically important in low-income countries with poor power supply, as well diesel power construction machines and industrial machines. It's important to note that even though most of the NO2 sources are from the outdoors, this outdoors contaminants could penetrate inside houses and became constant irritants to the households, making patients with pulmonary diseases more vulnerable [21]. Severe health effects of NO2 exposures would affect proximal airway causing worsened of cough with wheezes, causing increased in asthma exacerbations, leading to more hospital admissions. Constant exposure will eventually cause increased airway inflammation with remodeling of the airway, making it more severe with time. This patient will be escalating asthma treatments quickly without major relief and eventually will ne on advanced asthma treatments of this exposures are not recognized. There are multiple scientific studies that link decreased in pulmonary function such as diminished peak flows with higher exposure of N02. Avoidance and early recognition of improperly used heating devices and combustion devices is of greatest importance for avoidance [22]. Special attention to poorly vented placed, in which combustion products are been produced such as Nitrogen dioxide (NO2), carbon monoxide, Sulfur dioxide (SO2) and particulate matter as previously mentioned is key on the management of this patients.

3.4 Dust mites

Dust Mites are a worldwide problem in respiratory vulnerable patients. This are tiny organism that live in furniture's such as beddings, bed, soft toys, and clothing most of the time at people's homes. This organism is not airborne they live in soft and humid environments [23]. Dust mites most of the time become airborne with cleaning activities such as vacuum and dusting which organism will be mobilized and as other particulate matter react to nasal receptors and start the perpetuating sequela. Dust mite allergies can be detected with blood samples, for better preventive measures which the goal when recognizing exacerbating factors. Other preventive measures that will be discussed is the use of allergen proof mattress with pillowcases, close washing of bedding in a weakly basis, carpets and rugs management with high efficiency particulate air filter. The physiology of symptoms starts with indoor mites that are constantly feeding from death skin, that eventually will liberate allergens during that chemical process that will eventually lead to an asthma trigger, that most of the time will start with upper airway symptoms, with eventual bronchospasm due to airway hyperresponsiveness. It's important to recognize Dust mites because it's a strong allergen, difficult to take care of, and take meticulous weekly indoor management protocols for prevention of exacerbations. Asthma medications can help ameliorate dust mite reaction, but preventive measures with bedding cleaning, keeping beds with dust proof covers as well warm cleaning with higher degree temperature is the recommended range for adequate cleaning [24].

3.5 Cockroaches

Cockroaches are a worldwide populates pest with more than 3500 species known. They are most found in cities with highest urban population. Exposure to this indoor and outdoor pest, are well known causative agents of asthma and atopy respectively, and constant exposure this have been linked to increase asthma morbidity, which makes this environmental factors highly important in the recognition and management [25]. The cause of allergy and asthma exacerbations is been cause by proteins produced by cockroaches in which can be found in feces and body fluids of this animals. It's been stipulated that almost 60% of homes in the US have cockroaches, which is a big number comparing the high incidence of asthma and allergy, so we are continuously dealing with a difficult pest every day. There are several known cockroaches' species which are Blattella germanica and Periplaneta americana, which both produce the protein responsible for asthma triggers. Several proteins been recognized are Bla g 2(inactive aspartic proteinase), Bla g 4 (calycin) and Bla g 5 (glutathione-S-transferase) [26]. With these molecular recognized proteins, we can quantify exposure levels, which will eventually help in difficult to treat patient with asthma, in which exposure or triggers have not been recognized and subsequently avoided. Cockroaches induced allergic inflammation is the main driver in asthma exacerbations and difficult to manage asthma patients, this excreted particles from this organism can gain access to the upper respiratory tract through the nose and oral cavities with dislodgment into the lungs causing allergen epithelial damage. Cockroach allergy is diagnosed with crude extract via skin testing or direct measurement of serum specific IgE to this specific allergen, in this case cockroach. This serum levels can be use to recognized other multiple specific allergens. However, even though good sanitation and successful extermination actions are taken, sustained decrease in allergens levels is difficult to accomplish. It's important to recognized other environmental factors in this patient such as constant particulate matter exposure because air pollutants can increase the allergic effect of cockroaches and other indoor allergens with a synergistic relationship, a multidisciplinary approach for recognition is recommended to be effective in management.

3.6 Cats

There is a strong association between pet ownership and new onset asthma as well the development of allergic symptoms. Cats had been recognized as a major source of allergens for many years. They can produce numerous allergens that can trigger asthma symptoms. These allergens can be found in cats saliva, in which at the act of cats self-grooming its transfer to the skin, producing contact dermatitis changes as well can be inhaled in combination with cats dander causing asthma as well causes difficult to treat disease in patients with continuous exposure. Cats dander is another component of cats that comes from dead skin sweat glands that can suspend in the air consequently getting into the airways. As can be seen in other animal allergic sources component, cats urine can be the source of asthma, ligated with the protein Felis domesticus (Fel d 1) found in urine which can cause airway diseases as well [27]. Touching or inhaling these allergens causes overreaction of the immune system, leading to worsening of asthma symptoms. Asthma in adults differs from children in which atopy and exposure to aeroallergens are a determinant factor that could cause airway hyperresponsiveness [28]. Allergic asthma is a difficult to treat disease, however blood markers with specific IgE components which can be range from rFel d 1 which is a marker for severe asthma, and specifically indicates that is related to cats. Other components been found in asthma is rFel d 2, rFel d 4 and r Fel d7 by which its less specific for cats because it can be present in patients with dogs, horse and mice exposures [29, 30]. The best therapeutic option in this patient population is to avoid contact with animals specially cats or dogs, and very importantly to avoid indirect contact with areas that animals spent time. Keeping animals in the outdoor setting is appropriate, however allergens will remain in indoor spaces, by which aggressive hygiene needs to take part on the management.

3.7 Molds

Mold is a fungal growth that spread in surfaces, where most of the will be organic matter however it's not always the case. It can be found indoors and outdoors respectively, they will most of the time look for excess moisture places which is the most common cause of indoor mold environment. Molds are well recognized allergens related to asthma exacerbations, and most of the time will go not recognized [31]. Inhaling or contact with molds can cause allergic reactions, in which can trigger asthma symptoms, which can be manifested as sneezing, throat irritation, nasal stuffiness with runny nose and watery eyes, which are active signs of ongoing allergic process. Most of the patients will recognized this early symptom and could be able to attach specific interaction with the causing allergen, however molds are more difficult to be recognized. Most of the sources of mold in indoor settings will have water leaks associated with it, such as can be seen in air conditioners and leaks from outsource of water in close buildings. Molds not only can exacerbate asthma, but they are also well recognized factor of causing fatal respiratory conditions such as hypersensitivity pneumonitis which can be acute and could lead to respiratory failure [32]. There are several home situations even outdoors that needs to take in consideration when dealing with molds, and it's the existence of plumbing leaks, roof leaks and high humidity places, mostly indoors. Management of high-risk exposure places is important in occupational environmental, by which early detection in the setting of high suspiciousness is of great importance. Regular inspection of buildings, regular schedule air conditioning cleaning, adequate ventilation of close spaces and the importance of developing a indoor environment quality control group that will remain on top of this circumstances for adequate management [33]. Molds can produce spores which can be inhaled, that will produce allergic symptoms with upper airway predominance, this mold could weaken the natural defense mechanism o the airway that could lead to predisposition to colds and flu diseases. Special interest is been taken about molds in occupation setting environments, in which working personnel will became symptomatic in specific working areas and not at home places, in this special setting aggressive interrogation and evaluation is of most importance to prevent future exacerbations of lung diseases specially asthma.

3.8 Pollens

Pollen is the composition of tiny grains produced by plants for the purpose of fertilization. The wind is the main driver to spread the pollen to different areas, remaining most of the time suspended in the air. It is an important asthma allergen which could exacerbated allergic symptoms such as conjunctivitis, rhinitis and respiratory conditions [34]. Polinization periods are recognized as the peaks in pollen grains in the environment which remain suspended in the air causing allergic symptoms at inhalation. It had been recognized that pollen can be simultaneously combined with air pollution, increasing the changes of asthma and makes particles more easily to breath in. This makes polinization seasons challenging to physicians, making difficult to treat patients most vulnerable to this factor. Pollen season ranges from March to April respectively in which it can last up to 6 months [35]. There are multiple algorithmic maps which shows the percentage of pollen counts around the United States in which it can be characterize as low (0–2.4), low medium (2.5–4.8), medium (4.9–7.2), medium high (7.3–9.6) and high (9.7–12). It's important to understand that dry, windy days can cause allergy symptoms to get worse, however humid and rainy days can sometimes be beneficial to people with allergies. Physiology of this correlates making heavier pollen molecules making it most likely to stay on the ground.

3.9 Environmental tobacco smoke (ETS)

Environmental tobacco smoke is generated by the combustion of tobacco smoke. It is commonly emitted with combustion, which is actively exhale from the smoker. Tobacco smoke is composed of more than 4000 toxic compounds, most of them well known to have carcinogen effects [36]. There are two types of environmental tobacco smoke, which can be divided into side stream smoke which is the smoke from tobacco that is released from the end of a burning cigarette or tobacco pipe. Mainstream smoke refers to the smoke that is inhaled by a smoker that is actively exhaled to the environment and subsequently inhaled by a second person causing inhalation exposure. Side stream smoke is also of danger if prolonged exposure of time, side stream can persist affecting the smoker and not smoker in close rooms [37]. Several factors had been recognized that can affect the amount of side stream smoke which is humidity, temperature, open ventilation versus close ventilation and number of active smokers in the room. At this moment there is some data suggesting that second hand smoking can cause obstructive lung diseases as well however it's something that under investigation.

3.10 Outdoor air pollution

There are several groups of air pollutants which are ozone, particulate matter as previously discussed, sulfur dioxide, nitrogen dioxide, carbon monoxide and lead

Environmental Triggers of Asthma			
Mold and moisture	Environmental Tobacco Smoker	Gas Stoves	Viral Infections
Dust Mites	Hairspray/Personal Chemical Irritants	Wood Smoke	Sinus Inflammation
Cockroaches and Rodents	Air Conditioning	Outdoor Pollution/Particula te Matter	Emotions
Strong Odors/Perfumes	Food/Drinks	Nitrogen Dioxide/Sulfur Dioxide	Exercise
Weather/Cold Air	Grass	Molds	Medications
Animal Exposures	Cleaning Products	Workplace Exposure	Ozone
Pollen	Pesticides	Humidity	

Figure 7.
Environmental triggers of asthma.

respectively. There are multiple environmental triggers of asthma (**Figure 7**). Its Ozone the most recognized factor linked to asthma exacerbations, as well the cause of triggering asthma symptoms. Ozone forms in the air it's not visible, it cannot be smell or taste neither, but it can have strong health impact aggravating asthma symptoms, subsequently increasing use of medications, as well admissions to the hospital due to respiratory conditions. Ozone can be worse in patients with asthma, by which they will be more responsive to inflammation [38]. There are several studies comparing ambient ozone concentrations with increased asthma symptoms, as well risk of hospitalizations and decompensation. There is a positive correlation between severity of asthma and risk of ozone related effects. Traffic related pollutants are part of outdoor environmental factors as well diesel exhaust combustions.

4. Treatment, management and prevention

As we mentioned before, asthma is a common chronic disease characterized by episodic or persistent respiratory symptoms and airflow limitation, requiring ongoing and comprehensive treatment with the goal to reduce symptoms and minimize the risk of developments of exacerbations, and treatment side effects. The pathophysiology of the disease is complex and heterogeneous for which treatment is based on a stepwise approach and the management is control-based. This involves interactive cycle assessment where symptoms and risk factors are evaluated, adjustment of treatment and review of response in which patient preferences should also be taken into account. Anti-inflammatory treatment has been the mainstay of asthma management to reduce airway inflammation and help prevent symptoms; among these are the inhaled corticosteroids. For rapid relief of symptoms short-acting beta agonists (SABA) are the ones used to reduce airway bronchoconstriction causing relaxation of airway smooth muscles. The National and International guidelines have recommended SABA as the first line treatment for patients with mild asthma, since the Global Initiative for Asthma guideline (GINA) was first published in 1995, adopting the approach to control symptoms rather than the underlying condition. GINA was established by the WHO and NHLBI in 1993 to increase awareness about asthma and to improve asthma prevention and management through a coordinated worldwide effort. The SABA approach was initially thought to be due believing that asthma symptoms were related to bronchoconstriction rather than presence of a concomitant condition caused by airway inflammation.

GINA 2019 guideline review introduced substantial changes, adjusting asthma treatment for individual patients and adopting the concept of anti-inflammatory reliever in all degrees of severity as a crucial component in the management of the disease and efficacy of the treatment. The use of reliever medication (SABA) was placed as an addendum in the recommendations to be used in case the real treatment (the controller) failed to maintain disease control. As we know, SABA can effectively induce rapid symptom relief but are ineffective on the underlying inflammatory process. To achieve control, the intensity of the controller therapy was related to the disease severity with preferred controlled choice varying from low-dose inhaled corticosteroids (ICS)/long-acting bronchodilator (LABA), medium-dose ICS/LABA, up to high-dose ICS/LABA and with a SABA as the rescue medication. As a result of this patients with mild disease or mild symptoms were left without any anti-inflammatory treatment such as ICS and relying only on SABA rescue treatment. An important point to mention is one of the major limitations for control of asthma, which is poor adherence to therapy. A lot of patients seem to be administering inhaled medication only when asthma symptoms occur. In the absence of symptoms, patients perceive therapy unnecessary and avoid taking controlled medication. Therefore, when symptoms worsen, patients prefer to use reliever therapy which could result in overuse of SABA. An as seen in previous studies, there is evidence that suggest that overuse of beta-agonist alone is associated with risk of death from asthma, and at the same time with each exacerbation the risk of death also increases. Regular use of SABA, even for 1–2 weeks, is associated in increased airway hyper-responsiveness (AHR), reduced bronchodilator effect, increased allergic response and eosinophils [39].

Based on this evidence, in latest GINA 2022 guidelines treatment options are recommended in 5 Steps and divided in two tracks, to clarify how to step treatment up and down with the same reliever. First track which is the preferred strategy, is with the use of low-dose ICS/LABA (formoterol) as a reliever, introducing the single maintenance and reliever treatment (SMART). This strategy is the preferred due to evidence suggesting reduced risk of exacerbations compared with use of SABA only as a reliever, with similar symptoms control and lung function [40]. The SMART strategy containing the rapid-acting formoterol was recommended throughout GINA Steps based on solid evidence [41]. This recommendation continues since GINA 2019, where SABA as a reliever alone in STEP 1 was no longer recommended based on key studies SYGMA 1, SYGMA 2, Novel START and PRACTICAL [42, 43].

The second track, which is an alternative non-preferred strategy, is with the use of SABA as the reliever. This strategy is less effective in reducing exacerbations, however, continues to be used in case that therapy with low-dose ICS/LABA (Formoterol) is not possible. Also, it can be considered if patient has good adherence with their controller and has had no exacerbation in the last year. For patients who have asthma that remains uncontrolled after step 4 treatment should be referred for phenotypic assessment with or without add-on therapy. As mentioned before asthma is a complex and heterogeneous disease for which therapy should be individualized based on the underlying condition, presence or absence of allergy, and other coexisting conditions. In severe asthma or difficult-to-treat asthma, poor control can be linked to poor

Are there things in your environment that make your asthma worse?
Relevant environmental control and avoidance strategies - How to identify home, school or work exposures. - How to control house dust mites, animal exposure, adequate cleaning habits and tobacco exposure if applicable. - How to recognized dangerous environments that could lead to asthma ahead of time.
Recognition: Have you noticed anything in your environment that makes your asthma worse? - If Yes, consult your physician on ways to prevent them and how to diagnosed this exposures with clinical correlation.
Avoidance and Rescue Strategies Discussion and Plan with your physician.

Figure 8.
Relevant questions to identify environmental factors contributing to difficult to treat asthma.

adherence to medication, incorrect inhaler technique, and coexisting conditions, including exposure to allergens and irritants. Based on this the National Asthma Education Prevention Program (NAEPP) they recommended multicomponent allergen mitigation in sensitized individuals who have exposure to indoor allergen for pets. It was recommended to do integrated pest management alone, or as part of multi-core component intervention, and for dust mites that recommended using impermeable covers only as part of multicomponent intervention. Immunotherapy is recommended in mild to moderate allergic asthma but recommended using sub cutaneous immunotherapy. Also, important component of this therapy is to avoid any allergens or irritants that may trigger disease including smoke, dust mite, cockroach, animals, etc. Irritant or allergen sensitivity can also be determined by patient exposure and symptoms history, confirmed with skin or blood test. Leukotriene modifiers who have been used widely are mostly used especially in aspirin exacerbated respiratory disease and exercise-induced bronchial constriction who have been shown to have greater response.

When we are dealing with environmental and occupation factors, we need to categorize the patient and start the adequate therapy. The most important step is to make the diagnosis which can be made with peak flow changes in different environments of interest or investigated exposures. Changes in symptoms with changes in expiratory flow are classic in environmental exposures causing symptoms. Most of the patients will have recognized symptoms when exposed to the irritant or allergen. In patients that exposure is not clear, several algorithms of identification can be used with specific questions of daily life activities. Relevant questions to identify environmental factors (**Figure 8**).

5. Conclusion

As been discussed during this chapter, there are multiple environmental and occupation factors that are well known to cause asthma and worsening of asthma symptoms. Many triggers been recognized that can be divided into allergic and non allergic which is important at the moment of symptoms interrogation. A methodology approach and personalized approach need to be done for early and proper recognition of this factors. Educational programs on avoidance and recognition needs to be provided to the general population as well, education regarding common symptoms when dealing with this exposure which will eventually lead for better patient respiratory control and quality of life.

Conflict of interest

The authors declare no conflict of interest.

Author details

Christian Castillo Latorre*, Sulimar Morales Colon, Alba D. Rivera Diaz, Vanessa Fonseca Ferrer, Mariana Mercader Perez, Ilean Lamboy Hernandez, Luis Gerena Montano, William Rodriguez Cintron and Onix Cantres Fonseca
VA Caribbean Healthcare System, San Juan, Puerto Rico

*Address all correspondence to: ccl0332@gmail.com

IntechOpen

© 2022 The Author(s). Licensee IntechOpen. This chapter is distributed under the terms of the Creative Commons Attribution License (http://creativecommons.org/licenses/by/3.0), which permits unrestricted use, distribution, and reproduction in any medium, provided the original work is properly cited.

References

[1] Global Initiative for Asthma. Global Strategy for Asthma Management and Prevention. 2021. Available from: www.ginasthma.org.

[2] Boczkowski J, Murciano D, Pichot MH, Ferretti A, Pariente R, Milic-Emili J. Expiratory flow limitation in stable asthmatic patients during resting breathing. American Journal of Respiratory and Critical Care Medicine. 1997;**156**(3 Pt 1):752-757. DOI: 10.1164/ajrccm.156.3.9609083

[3] Difficult To Treat & Severe Asthma in Adolescent and Adult Patients. Diagnosis and Management. A GINA Pocket Guide for Health Professionals. GINA Guidelines. V2.0 April 2019

[4] Global Initiative for Asthma. Difficult-to-Treat & Severe Asthama. GINA Pocket Guide. Global Initiative for Asthma; 2021

[5] Chabra R, Gupta M. Allergic and Environmental Induced Asthma. Treasure Island (FL): StatPearls Publishing; 2021

[6] Martinez FD. Genes, environments, development and asthma: A reappraisal. The European Respiratory Journal. 2007;**29**(1):179-184. DOI: 10.1183/09031936.00087906

[7] Blanc PD, Toren K. How much adult asthma can be attributed to occupational factors? The American Journal of Medicine. 1999;**107**(6):580-587. DOI: 10.1016/S0002-9343(99)00307-1

[8] Rondinelli RD, Genovese E, Katz RT, Mayer TG, Mueller KL, Ranavaya MI, et al. The Pulmonary System. Sixth ed. AMA Guides to the Evaluation of Permanent Impairment. American Medical Association AMA; 2022. p. 2022

[9] Perlman DM, Maier LA. Occupational lung disease. Medical Clinics of North America. 2019;**103**(3):535-548

[10] Gautier C, Lecam MT, Basses S, Pairon JC, Andujar P. Définition de l'asthme en relation avec le travail et ses conséquences sociales et professionnelles chez l'adulte et l'adolescent [A definition of work-related asthma and its social and occupational consequences in adults and teenagers]. Revue des Maladies Respiratoires. 2021;**38**(9):914-935. DOI: 10.1016/j.rmr.2021.09.006

[11] Nordman H. Occupational asthma—Time for prevention. Scandinavian Journal of Work, Environment & Health. 1994;**20**:108-115

[12] Maestrelli P, Henneberger PK, Tarlo S, Mason P, Boschetto P. Causes and phenotypes of work-related asthma. International Journal of Environmental Research and Public Health. 2020;**17**(13):4713. DOI: 10.3390/ijerph17134713

[13] Vandenplas O, Godet J, Hurdubaea L, Rifflart C, Suojalehto H, Wiszniewska M, et al. Are high- and low-molecular-weight sensitizing agents associated with different clinical phenotypes of occupational asthma? Allergy. 2019;**74**:261-272. DOI: 10.1111/all.13542

[14] Global Initiative for Asthma. Global strategy for asthma management and prevention. Available from: https://ginasthma.org/ [Accessed: March 16, 2022]

[15] Tan DJ, Walters EH, Perret JL, et al. Clinical and functional differences between early-onset and late-onset adult asthma: A population-based Tasmanian longitudinal health study. Thorax. 2016;**71**:981

[16] Stanojevic S, Kaminsky DA, Miller M, et al. ERS/ATS technical standard on interpretive strategies for routine lung function tests. The European Respiratory Journal. 2021;**60**:2101499

[17] Breysse PN, Diette GB, Matsui EC, Butz AM, Hansel NN, McCormack MC. Indoor air pollution and asthma in children. Proceedings of the American Thoracic Society. 2010;**7**(2):102-106. DOI: 10.1513/pats.200908-083RM

[18] Pope CA 3rd, Dockery DW. Health effects of fine particulate air pollution: Lines that connect. Journal of the Air & Waste Management Association (1995). 2006;**56**(6):709-742. DOI: 10.1080/10473289.2006.10464485

[19] Takizawa H. Impacts of particulate air pollution on asthma: Current understanding and future perspectives. Recent Patents on Inflammation & Allergy Drug Discovery. 2015; **9**(2):128-135. DOI: 10.2174/1872213x09666150623110714

[20] Singh N, Singh S. Interstitial lung diseases and air pollution: Narrative review of literature. Pulmonary Therapy. 2021;**7**:89-100. DOI: 10.1007/s41030-021-00148-7

[21] Sunyer J, Basagaña X, Belmonte J, et al. Effect of nitrogen dioxide and ozone on the risk of dying in patients with severe asthma. Thorax. 2002;**57**:687-693

[22] J. Gillespie-Bennett, N. Pierse, K. Wickens, J. Crane, P. Howden-Chapman, and the Housing Heating and Health Study Research Team. The respiratory health effects of nitrogen dioxide in children with asthma. European Respiratory Journal, 2011, 38 (2) 303-309; DOI: 10.1183/09031936.00115409.

[23] Milián E, Díaz AM. Allergy to house dust mites and asthma. Puerto Rico Health Sciences Journal. Mar 2004;**23**(1):47-57

[24] Wilson JM, Platts-Mills TAE. Home environmental interventions for house dust mite. The Journal of Allergy and Clinical Immunology Practice. 2018;**6**(1):1-7. DOI: 10.1016/j.jaip.2017.10.003

[25] Do DC, Zhao Y, Gao P. Cockroach allergen exposure and risk of asthma. Allergy. 2016;**71**:463-474

[26] Pomés A, Chapman MD, Vailes LD, Blundell TL, Dhanaraj V. Cockroach allergen Bla g 2: Structure, function, and implications for allergic sensitization. American Journal of Respiratory and Critical Care Medicine. 2002;**165**(3):391-397. DOI: 10.1164/ajrccm.165.3.2104027

[27] Kelly LA, Erwin EA, Platts-Mills TA. The indoor air and asthma: The role of cat allergens. Current Opinion in Pulmonary Medicine. 2012;**18**(1):29-34. DOI: 10.1097/MCP.0b013e32834db10d

[28] Baxi SN, Phipatanakul W. The role of allergen exposure and avoidance in asthma. Adolescent Medicine: State of the Art Reviews. 2010;**21**(1):57-71

[29] Quirce S, Dimich-Ward H, Chan H, Ferguson A, Becker A, Manfreda J, et al. Major cat allergen (Fel d I) levels in the homes of patients with asthma and their relationship to sensitization to cat dander. Annals of Allergy, Asthma & Immunology. 1995;**75**(4):325-330

[30] Bonnet B, Messaoudi K, Jacomet F, et al. An update on molecular cat allergens: Fel d 1 and what else? Chapter 1: Fel d 1, the major cat allergen. Allergy, Asthma and Clinical Immunology. 2018;**14**:14. DOI: 10.1186/s13223-018-0239-8

[31] Ma Y, Tian G, Tang F, et al. The link between mold sensitivity and asthma

severity in a cohort of northern Chinese patients. Journal of Thoracic Disease. 2015;7(4):585-590. DOI: 10.3978/j.issn.2072-1439.2015.01.04

[32] Denis Caillaud, Benedicte Leynaert, Marion Keirsbulck, Rachel Nadif, on behalf of the mould ANSES working group. Indoor mould exposure, asthma and rhinitis: Findings from systematic reviews and recent longitudinal studies. European Respiratory Review, 2018;**27**:170137; DOI: 10.1183/16000617.0137-2017.

[33] OSHA. Preventing Mold Related Problems in the Indoor Workplace. A Guide for Building Owners, Managers and Occupants. U.S. Department of Labor Occupational Safety and Health Administration OSHA. Occupational and Safety Health Administration; 2006. Available from: www.osha.gov

[34] Osborne NJ, Alcock I, Wheeler BW, Hajat S, Sarran C, Clewlow Y, et al. Pollen exposure and hospitalization due to asthma exacerbations: Daily time series in a European city. International Journal of Biometeorology. 2017;**61**(10):1837-1848. DOI: 10.1007/s00484-017-1369-2

[35] Singh N, Singh U, Singh D, Daya M, Singh V. Correlation of pollen counts and number of hospital visits of asthmatic and allergic rhinitis patients. Lung India. 2017;**34**(2):127-131. DOI: 10.4103/0970-2113.201313

[36] Baker RR, Proctor CJ. The origins and properties of environmental tobacco smoke. Environment International. 1990;**16**(3):231-245. DOI: 10.1016/0160-4120(90)90117-O

[37] Löfroth G. Environmental tobacco smoke: Overview of chemical composition and genotoxic components. Mutation Research/Genetic Toxicology. 1989;**222**(2):73-80. DOI: 10.1016/0165-1218(89)90021-9

[38] Khatri SB, Holguin FC, Ryan PB, Mannino D, Erzurum SC, Teague WG. Association of ambient ozone exposure with airway inflammation and allergy in adults with asthma. The Journal of Asthma. 2009;**46**(8):777-785

[39] Suissa S, Ernst P, Benayoun S, Baltzan M, Cai B. Low-dose inhaled corticosteroids and the prevention of death from asthma. The New England Journal of Medicine. 2000;**343**(5):332-336

[40] Pauwels RA, Löfdahl CG, Postma DS, Tattersfield AE, O'Byrne P, Barnes PJ, et al. Effect of inhaled formoterol and budesonide on exacerbations ofasthma. The New England Journal of Medicine. 1997;**337**(20):1405-1411

[41] Global Initiative for Asthma. Global Strategy for Asthma Management and Prevention. Global Initiative for Asthma GINA guidelines; 2017. Available from: http://www.ginasthma.org [Accessed: June 1, 2019].

[42] Bateman ED, Reddel HK, O'Byrne PM, Barnes PJ, Zhong N, Keen C, et al. As-needed budesonide–formoterol versus maintenance budesonide in mild asthma. The New England Journal of Medicine. 2018;**378**(20):1877-1887

[43] O'Byrne PM, FitzGerald JM, Bateman ED, Barnes PJ, Zhong N, Keen C, et al. Inhaled combined budesonide-formoterol as needed in mild asthma. The New England Journal of Medicine. 2018;**378**(20):1865-1876

Chapter 5

Effect of Family Education on Clinical Outcomes in Children with Asthma: A Review

Maha Dardouri, Manel Mallouli, Jihene Sahli, Chekib Zedini, Jihene Bouguila and Ali Mtiraoui

Abstract

Childhood asthma still imposes an enormous burden on children and their families. To the best of our knowledge, no study reviewed the literature on the effect of family asthma education on major asthma outcomes. This study aimed to explore the effect of family education programs on major asthma outcomes in children. Quasi-experimental studies and randomized controlled trials were conducted among children with asthma aged 6–18 years and their parents were included. Pub Med, Science Direct, and Trip databases were used to extract data published in English from 2010 to 2021. Twenty-two studies were reported in this review. It was demonstrated that family empowerment interventions were effective in improving the quality of life of children and their parents, asthma symptom control, and pulmonary function. Family education that was specific to medication improved medication adherence, inhalation technique, and asthma control. Family asthma education enhanced asthma management and family functioning. This approach should be a cornerstone of pediatric asthma therapy. It helps health care professionals to build a strong connection and trustful relationship with children with asthma and their families.

Keywords: asthma, child, family, patient education, disease management

1. Introduction

Asthma is a serious childhood issue that still imposes an enormous burden on children, their families, and health care systems [1]. Currently, 339 million people worldwide suffer from asthma, and approximately 14% of children are affected [2]. In 2019, asthma caused 2.29% of total disability adjusted life years and 3.76% of years lived with disability in children with asthma aged 5–14 years worldwide [3]. Besides, pediatric asthma affects the parents through the loss of productivity at the workplace and family disruption [1, 4].

The Global Atlas of Asthma stated that asthma is one of the main causes of hospitalization in children [5]. Additionally, a recent study noted that children and adolescents with asthma had a higher number of outpatient and emergency department (ED) visits in comparison with non-asthmatic children [6]. The lack of asthma control can place severe limits on the daily life of children and is sometimes fatal. Treatment and effective management of asthma can save lives [7]. Patient education and self-management plans have been convincingly shown to reduce exacerbations requiring hospitalization [5]. Besides, a growing emphasis has been on involving families in health care and assessing their needs. Family education consists of the active involvement of the child and his or her parent in the process of chronic disease management and treatment [8, 9].

A recent systematic review examined the effectiveness of school- and community-based nurse-led educational interventions on asthma management for school-age children and their parents [10]. This literature review included eight studies published from 2014 to 2016, which is a limited sample. It reported that school- and community-based interventions led by nurses improved knowledge and skills related to asthma self-management in school-age children with asthma and their parents. Furthermore, Walter and colleagues systematically reviewed the effect of school-based family asthma education programs on QOL and asthma exacerbations in children with asthma aged 5–18 years. This review reported a limited number of randomized control trials (n = 6) published from 2004 to 2010. It revealed that school-based family asthma educational programs for children and their caregivers can have a positive effect on QOL and asthma management of children with asthma [11].

Numerous studies assessed the impact of family education on asthma major outcomes. The findings of these interventions were controversial. This study aimed to report results from recent studies on the effectiveness of family education on clinical outcomes in children with asthma.

2. Methods

2.1 Study design

This was a literature review of randomized and non-randomized controlled studies, which assessed the effectiveness of family asthma educational interventions on asthma outcomes. A regional Institutional Review Board approved the study under the approval number DEFMS 01/2018.

2.2 Sources of information

The data search was carried out using three electronic databases: PubMed, ScienceDirect, and Trip database. Data collection was conducted from January to December 2021. Studies identified in the references of the selected articles, and that met the inclusion criteria were included in this review (**Figure 1**).

2.3 Search strategies

The keywords used were: asthma, child, adolescent, caregivers, quality of life, education, and disease management.

These terms were combined via the Boolean switch statement "AND" and "OR", as following: (("Asthma"[Mesh]) AND "Child"[Mesh]) AND "Quality of Life"[Mesh]; ((("Asthma"[Mesh]) AND "Disease Management"[Mesh])

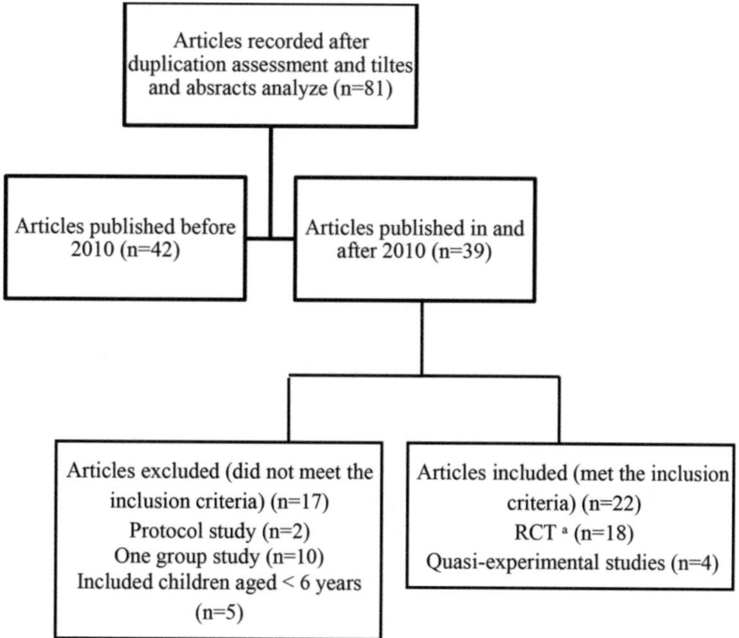

Figure 1.
The studies' selection procedure. [a]RCT: Randomized controlled trials.

AND "Child"[Mesh]) AND "Caregivers"[Mesh]; (((("Asthma"[Mesh]) AND "Child"[Mesh]) AND "Adolescent"[Mesh]) AND "Education" [Subheading]; (((("Asthma/nursing"[Majr] OR "Asthma/rehabilitation"[Majr] OR "Asthma/therapy"[Majr])) AND ("Patient Education as Topic/education"[Majr] OR "Patient Education as Topic/methods"[Majr] OR "Patient Education as Topic/organization and administration"[Majr])) AND "Family"[Mesh] AND "Child"[Mesh].

Randomized controlled trials and quasi-experimental studies published in English from 2010 to December 2021 were considered.

2.4 Selection criteria of the studies

Studies were primarily selected based on the titles and abstracts. After the exclusion of duplicates, studies were assessed according to the established inclusion criteria. Included studies were quasi-experimental studies or randomized controlled trials conducted in children with asthma aged between 6 and 18 years and their parents, and published (or accepted for publication) in English from January 2010 to December 2021. Abstracts and research protocols were excluded.

2.5 Data extraction

For each study included in this literature review, the following variables were identified: country and year of publication, study design, study groups, follow-up assessment, intervention approach, intervention duration, number of sessions, duration of each session, theoretical framework (if applicable), and clinical outcomes and their measurement tools.

3. Results

3.1 Selection of the studies

After removing duplicates, 81 articles were screened. Forty-two articles were removed since they were published before 2010. After the analysis of the full-text articles, 17 articles were excluded since they did not meet the inclusion criteria. Finally, 22 articles were included in this literature review.

3.2 Characteristics of the included studies

Table 1 shows that 9 studies were randomized controlled trials (RCT). The sample sizes of the reviewed studies ranged from 14 to 167 children with asthma, with a total of 1087 participants. The major target group of the educational interventions was asthmatic school-aged children and their families [13, 15–25]. Some studies included teachers [13], and asthma physicians [20]. Most of the educational sessions were conducted in groups. The duration of sessions varied between 30 and 120 minutes. The assessment time ranged from 2 weeks to 12 months.

The topics discussed in almost 90% of the educational sessions were asthma pathophysiology, triggers identification, symptoms recognition, effective response during exacerbations, asthma action plan, types of asthma medications and their correct use, and communication with care providers [16–25].

Five interventions were conducted by the research team of the trial [16–18, 22, 25]. Other interventions were carried out by a multidisciplinary team [24], and certified educators of asthma [15, 20].

Table 2 shows the outcomes assessed in each study and their assessment tools. The Pediatric Asthma Quality of Life Questionnaire and the Pediatric Asthma Caregiver Quality of Life Questionnaire were used to assess the QOL of children and their parents in all studies respectively. Different tools were used for symptoms control assessment. The Asthma Control Test (ACT) was commonly used.

3.3 Impact of educational interventions on asthma-related health outcomes

3.3.1 Quality of life

As shown in **Table 2**, five studies assessed the QOL of children with asthma, and three studies assessed the QOL of parents. One RCT [25] and two quasi-experimental studies [16, 17] referred to family empowerment in school-age children with asthma and their parents. Improved QOL scores were observed after implementing family empowerment interventions in Tunisia, Egypt, and Iran. Furthermore, the "Healthy Breathing Program" implemented by Grover and colleagues in children with asthma aged 7–12 years and their parents in India led to a significant improvement in the QOL scores of parents at six-month follow-up in the intervention group ($p < .001$) [18]. Similarly, the self-care education program contributed to improved QOL scores of children in Iran [23]. Montalbano et al. conducted a therapeutic asthma education that combines a multidisciplinary education with a smartphone application in school-age children with asthma and their parents in Italy. The program contributed to higher scores of QOL in the intervention and the control group at the three-month follow-up (Intervention group, $p = .014$; Control group, $p = .046$) [24].

The first author, year, country	Study design	Target population	Study groups	Follow-up assessment	Intervention approach	Intervention duration	Number of sessions	Duration of each session	Theory
Clark et al., 2010 [12], USA	RCT	Preteen students (5th to 8th grade)	Open airways at school (n = 468); open airways at school + peer asthma action (n = 416); control n = 408)	12 months 24 months	School-based, group	6 weeks	6	60 min	NA
McGhan et al., 2010 [13], Canada	RCT	Children aged 6–13 years (2nd to 5th grade), their parents, and teachers	The roaring adventures of puff (n = 104); usual care (n = 162)	6 months 12 months	School-based, group	NA	6 (children); 1 (parent/teacher)	45–60 min (children) 2 h (parent/teacher)	The social cognitive theory
Mosnaim et al., 2011 [14], USA	RCT	Youth (8–12 years) Teenagers (13–18 years)	FAN youth curriculum (n = 275), control (n = 69); FAN teen curriculum (n = 141), control (n = 51)	Posttest	School-based, group	4 consecutive school days	4	45 min	NA
USA	RCT	Adolescents aged 14–16 years (9th to 10th grade), their medical providers	Asthma self-management for adolescents (n = 175); control (n = 170)	6 months 12 months	School-based, group, and tailored individual	8 weeks (group) 5 weeks (individual)	3 (group) At least 1/week (individual)	45–60 min	The social cognitive theory

The first author, year, country	Study design	Target population	Study groups	Follow-up assessment	Intervention approach	Intervention duration	Number of sessions	Duration of each session	Theory
Celano et al., 2012 [15], USA	RCT	Children aged 8–13 years	Home-based family intervention (n = 23); enhanced treatment as usual (n = 20)	Posttest 6 months	Home-based, Individual	4 months	4–6	NA	NA
USA	RCT	Children aged 8–12 years	Modified open airways at school (n = 15); control (n = 17)	3 weeks 6 weeks	School-based, Group	3 weeks	3	90 min	NA
Canada	RCT	1316 Children aged 6–9 years and their families	The roaring adventures of puff; control	2 months 12 months	School-based, group	NA	6	45–60	The social cognitive theory
USA	RCT	Children of 9th to 12th grade (mean age of 15.6)	Tailored web-based program (n = 204); generic asthma websites (n = 218)	6 months 12 months	School-based, group	6 months	4	15–30	Behavioral theories
Payrovee et al., 2014 [16], Iran	Quasi-experimental	Children aged 7–11 years and their parents	Family empowerment intervention (n = 14); usual treatment (n = 16)	2 weeks	Family-based, group	4 weeks	4	2 h	NA

The first author, year, country	Study design	Target population	Study groups	Follow-up assessment	Intervention approach	Intervention duration	Number of sessions	Duration of each session	Theory
Fouda et al., 2015 [17], Egypt	Quasi-experimental	Children age 6–12 years and their parents	Family empowerment intervention (n = 23); usual care (n = 24)	2 weeks	Family-based, group	2 weeks	2	NA	NA
Grover et al. [18], India	RCT	Children aged 7–12 years and their parents	Healthy breathing program (n = 24); usual care (n = 16)	1 month 6 months	Individual parent-child pair	NA	1	1 h	Pedagogical principles
Arikan-Ayyildiz et al., 2016 [19], Turkey	RCT	Children age 6–12 years and their parents	Asthma education program (n = 26); usual care (n = 21)	1 month 3 months	Group	NA	1	1 h	NA
Canino et al., 2016 [20], Puerto Rico	RCT	Children with a mean age of 8.3, their families, and asthma physician	CALMA-plus (child, parent, physician) (n = 167); CALMA (child, parent) (n = 164)	6, 12, and 18 months	Home-based, individual	NA	2	NA	The social cognitive theory

The first author, year, country	Study design	Target population	Study groups	Follow-up assessment	Intervention approach	Intervention duration	Number of sessions	Duration of each session	Theory
Yeh et al., 2016 [21], Taiwan	RCT	Children aged 6–12 years and their families	Asthma family empowerment program + self-management intervention (n = 34); self-management intervention (n = 31)	3 months 1 year	Family-based	16 weeks	4	50 min	Freire's empowerment theory
Australia	RCT	Children aged 6–16 years	Electronic monitoring devices with reminder alarms (n = 47); electronic monitoring devices without reminder alarms (n = 42)	3, 6, 9, and 12 months	Individual	NA	1	NA	NA
Kashaninia et al., 2018 [22], Iran	Quasi-experimental	Children aged 6–12 years and their parents	Family empowerment intervention (n = 14); usual treatment (n = 16)	2 weeks	Family-based, group	4 weeks	4	2 h	NA
Mosenzadeh et al., 2018 [23], Iran	Quasi-experimental	Children aged 8–11 years and their parents	Self-care education (n = 35); usual treatment (n = 35)	8 weeks	Family-based, group	NA	4	45 min	NA

The first author, year, country	Study design	Target population	Study groups	Follow-up assessment	Intervention approach	Intervention duration	Number of sessions	Duration of each session	Theory
USA	RCT	Children aged 8–14 years, their caregivers, and school nurses	Telemedicine asthma education intervention (n = 180); usual care (n = 183)	3, and 6 months	School-based Individual (children) Group (caregivers and nurses)	5–9 weeks	5 (children) 2 (caregivers) 1 (nurses)	30–45 min (children) 60–90 min (caregivers and nurses)	NA
Netherlands	RCT	Adolescents aged 12–18 years	Interactive mobile health intervention (n = 87); usual care (n = 147)	6 months	Mobile phone application Individual	6 months	All-time during 6 months	All-time during 6 months	NA
Montalbano et al., 2019 [24], Italy	RCT	Children aged 6–11 years and their families	Mobile phone application and multidisciplinary education (n = 25); mobile application (n = 25)	1 month, 2, and 3 months	m-health program Group	3 months	3	30–60 min	NA
Dardouri et al., 2020, 2021 [25, 26], Tunisia	RCT	Children aged 7–17 years and their parents	Family empowerment program (n = 34) Usual care education (n = 34)	12 months	Family-centered care Group	2 months	4	60 min	Family empowerment model

RCT: Randomized Controlled Trial; NA: not available.

Table 1.
Description of the characteristics of family asthma educational interventions.

First author, year, country	Child's QOL	Parent's QOL	Asthma symptom control	Lung function	ED visit/ hospitalization	Adherence to treatment	Inhalation technique
Clark et al., 2010 [12], USA	Pediatric Asthma Quality of Life Questionnaire (PAQLQ)		Series of questions about the frequency of specific asthma symptoms in the past year during the day and at night				
McGhan et al., 2010 [13], Canada	PAQLQ				Number of ED visits in past year		
Mosnaim et al., 2011 [14], USA							The 8-item FAN Spacer Checklist
USA	PAQLQ		Number of symptom days and nights awoken in the last 2 weeks		Number of acute medical and ED visits, hospitalization		
Celano et al. 2012 [15], USA			Number of symptom days in last 2 weeks		Number of ED visits and hospitalizations in the past year		Metered dose inhaler checklist
USA	PAQLQ		Child Asthma Control Test	SpiroUSB portable spirometry machine			
Canada	PAQLQ				Number of urgent visits		Checklist
USA			Number of symptom days and nights		Number of ED visits		
Payrovee et al., 2014 [16], Iran	PAQLQ						
Fouda et al., 2015 [17], Egypt	PAQLQ	PACQLQ					

First author, year, country	Child's QOL	Parent's QOL	Asthma symptom control	Lung function	ED visit/ hospitalization	Adherence to treatment	Inhalation technique
Grover et al., 2015 [18], India		PACQL	Asthma Control Questionaire			Self-reported adherence	MD, Lupihaler and Rotahaler checklists
Arikan-Ayyildiz et al., 2016 [19], Turkey			Asthma Control Test		Number of ED visits and hospitalizations		
Canino et al., 2016 [20], Puerto Rico			Symptom days and nights		Number of ED visits and hospitalizations		
Yeh et al., 2016 [21], Taiwan			Self-reported asthma symptoms	Portable Spirometer			
Australia	Mini PAQLQ		Asthma Control Questionnaire	Spirometry test	Number of ED visits	Number of daily doses taken	
Kashaninia et al., 2018 [22], Iran			Asthma Control Test				
Mosenzadeh et al., 2018 [23], Iran	PAQLQ						
USA	PedsQL 3.0 PAQLQ		Symptom free days in past 2 weeks	Spirometry test			
Netherlands	PAQLQ					Medication Adherence Report Scale	

First author, year, country	Child's QOL	Parent's QOL	Asthma symptom control	Lung function	ED visit/ hospitalization	Adherence to treatment	Inhalation technique
Montalbano et al., 2019 [24], Italy	PAQLQ		Asthma Control Test	Portable spirometer		Medication Adherence Report Scale	
Dardouri et al., 2020 [25], Tunisia	PAQLQ	PACQLQ		Spirometry test using ZAN 100 machine			
Dardouri et al., 2021 [26], Tunisia			GINA guidelines		Number of ED visits and hospitalizations	Number of doses used weekly	Inhaler checklist

ED: emergency department; PAQLQ: Pediatric Asthma Quality of Life Questionnaire.

Table 2.
Asthma outcomes and measurement tools used by the studies included in the systematic review.

3.3.2 Asthma symptom control

It was demonstrated that family education contributed to a significant decrease in asthma symptoms days and nights [15, 18, 20]. Indeed, family empowerment interventions were significantly effective in reducing asthma symptoms, such as coughing, wheezing, and dyspnea ($p < .0001$) [21], and improving asthma symptom control in school-age children ($p < .001$) [22, 26, 27]. Besides, the m-Health program of Montalbano et al. was effective in improving the Child-Asthma Control Test scores ($p = .0089$) in the intervention group [24].

3.3.3 Pulmonary function

Two family empowerment interventions led to a significant improvement in pulmonary function parameters, including forced vital capacity (FVC) and forced expiratory volume in 1 s (FEV1) ($p < .05$) [21, 25]. Moreover, Montalbano et al. revealed that the m-health program combined with multidisciplinary education contributed to a better performance of forced expiratory maneuvers [24].

3.3.4 Acute health care utilization

The *"Roaring Adventures of Puff"* program incorporated a multitude of childhood educational approaches based on theory and evidence of factors that influence a child's motivation and self-efficacy [13]. This school-based program targeted the children and their support community (parents, peers, and teachers). After a 12-month follow-up, the number of unscheduled doctors and ED visits due to asthma was reduced in the experimental and the control group. However, three child-parent education programs did not show a significant difference in ED visits and hospitalizations between the intervention and the control group at follow-up [19, 20, 26].

3.3.5 Medication use: Inhaler technique and adherence.

A medication education program for children and their parents contributed to an improvement in inhaler technique and self-reported adherence to the prescribed medication [18]. Besides, Celano et al. showed that, at follow-up, a greater proportion of children who received a home-based family intervention demonstrated adequate technique as compared to children in the usual care group (84%; 44%; $p = .019$ respectively) [15]. A recent RCT showed that a six-month family empowerment intervention improved inhalation techniques in children with asthma [26]. However, the same intervention was not effective in enhancing medication adherence.

4. Discussion

The family, as the core of society, is responsible for providing adequate care for children. Besides, it should have correct information and perception of the child's disease [28]. According to Piaget's theory, school-aged children (7 to less than 12) gain the ability to solve concrete problems [25]. For that, they can manage and control asthma by themselves and with their parents' supervision through education and support. The fact of being responsible for asthma management as a school-age child is a huge development, which provides strength and command over the disease. The National Heart, Lung and Blood Institute (NHLBI), and the Global Initiative for Asthma (GINA) strictly emphasize educating asthmatic children, their parents, and health care professionals [1, 29]. Family education has a crucial role in empowering children and their families to effectively control and manage asthma. Evidence supported pediatric nurses to educate children with asthma and their families [8, 9]. The British guideline on asthma management suggested that family therapy may be a useful adjunct to medication use in children with asthma [30].

In this study, we reviewed the characteristics and the impact of family education on asthma outcomes. The reported asthma clinical outcomes were QOL, asthma symptom control, pulmonary function, ED use/hospitalization, medication adherence, and inhalation technique. This literature review revealed that home- and clinic-based family education was significantly effective in enhancing the QOL of children with asthma and their parents and asthma symptom control. Five family interventions improved pulmonary function, medication adherence, and inhalation technique [15, 18, 21, 24, 26]. One family education program reduced ED use [13].

Indeed, family interventions are needed to develop empowerment skills in families to take care of asthmatic children [21, 25]. The literature revealed that family empowerment education based on empowerment theories enhanced the QOL of children and parents, asthma symptom control, and pulmonary function in asthmatic children, as well as reduced parental stress [16, 17, 21, 22, 25]. Moreover, the use of predetermined open-ended communication, meaningful learning, art therapy, problem-solving, and goal setting principles was advantageous for better medication use, parent's QOL, and asthma symptom control [18]. Besides, the multidisciplinary intervention that included a pediatrician, a pediatric pulmonologist, a pediatric psychologist, and two experts in the field of Information and Communication Technologies-based tools had a crucial role in improving the QOL of children, forced expiratory maneuvers, and asthma symptom control [24].

The synthesis of the literature demonstrated that it is beneficial to educate children and their parents about the different asthma aspects in group sessions at home, school, or in clinical settings. Asthma aspects can include asthma pathophysiology, triggers identification, symptoms recognition, effective response during exacerbations, asthma action plan, types of asthma medications and their correct use, and communication with care providers. The interventions must be age-appropriate, culture-tailored, and well-designed to satisfy the unmet health care needs of families of children with asthma. These data suggested that family interventions can promote the health of asthmatic children in diverse settings. Furthermore, this study revealed that family asthma educational interventions were widely and successfully implemented in lower- and upper-middle income countries, including Tunisia, India, Egypt, Iran, and Turkey [31].

This literature review presented several limitations. First, articles published in languages other than English were not considered. Second, only three databases were used for data search. Due to these facts, some of the relevant articles may not be included in this literature review. Besides, half of the studies included (11 of 22 studies) had small samples, which can limit the generalizability of the results. However, this literature review reported recent interventions in detail. The practice implication for pediatric nurses was noticeable and fitted the guidelines of the National Heart, Lung and Blood Institute, and the Global Initiative for Asthma.

5. Application to practice

Pediatric nurses have a crucial role in promoting family asthma interventions. They are well-positioned to empower families of children with asthma to achieve optimal asthma control. Through family interventions, pediatric nurses can build a strong connection and trusting relationship with children with asthma and their families. Such strategies can improve asthma control and reduce ED use [13, 21, 22]. In family interventions, pediatric nurses should provide families of asthmatic children with unmet health care needs, supportive communication, correct use of medication, and effective ways of exacerbation prevention. Family interventions supported the active involvement and collaboration of families in the asthma therapeutic regimen of their affected children.

6. Conclusions

Asthma education is a key component of asthma management. Well-established family interventions can promote the health of children and improve the QOL of parents, when conducted at home, school, or in a clinic. The current review added to existent literature that family asthma education was effective in improving major asthma outcomes, including QOL, asthma symptom control, pulmonary function, and inhalation technique. This type of intervention was highly recommended to be applied by pediatric nurses. Scant family interventions reduced ED use and enhanced medication adherence. Family intervention associated with innovative technologies such as artificial intelligence may help children and families to better adhere to their medication and manage asthma crises to reduce ED visits. New asthma research should assess the effectiveness of family education associated with artificial intelligence on medication adherence and ED visits.

Conflict of interest

The authors declare no conflict of interest.

Author details

Maha Dardouri[1*], Manel Mallouli[1,2], Jihene Sahli[1,2], Chekib Zedini[1,2], Jihene Bouguila[3] and Ali Mtiraoui[1,2]

1 Faculty of Medicine of Sousse "Ibn El Jazzar", Research Laboratory "Quality of Care and Management of Maternal Health Services" (LR12ES03), University of Sousse, Sousse, Tunisia

2 Faculty of Medicine of Sousse Department of Community and Family Medicine, "Ibn El Jazzar", University of Sousse, Sousse, Tunisia

3 Department of Pediatrics, Farhat Hached University Hospital, Sousse, Tunisia

*Address all correspondence to: maha.dardouri@famso.u-sousse.tn

IntechOpen

© 2022 The Author(s). Licensee IntechOpen. This chapter is distributed under the terms of the Creative Commons Attribution License (http://creativecommons.org/licenses/by/3.0), which permits unrestricted use, distribution, and reproduction in any medium, provided the original work is properly cited. (cc) BY

References

[1] Global Initiative for Asthma. Global Strategy for Asthma Management and Prevention. 2019. Available from: https://ginasthma.org/reports/. [Accessed: July 01, 2019]

[2] Global Asthma Network. The Global Asthma Report. 2018. Available from: http://www.globalasthmareport.org/burden/burden.php. [Accessed: May 08, 2020]

[3] Institute for Health Metrics and Evaluation. Global Burden Disease. 2019. Available from: https://vizhub.healthdata.org/gbd-compare/. [Accessed: November 03, 2020]

[4] Ferrante G, La Grutta S. The burden of pediatric asthma. Frontiers in Pediatrics. 2018;**6**:186

[5] Akdis CA, Agache I. Global Atlas of Asthma. 2013. Available from: https://www.allergique.org/IMG/Global_Atlas_of_Asthma.pdf

[6] Nunes C, Pereira AM, Morais-Almeida M. Asthma costs and social impact. Asthma Research and Practice. 2017;**3**:1-11

[7] World Health Organization. Asthma. 2019. Available from: https://www.who.int/news-room/q-a-detail/asthma [Accessed: April 30, 2020]

[8] Divecha CA, Tullu MS, Jadhav DU. Parental knowledge and attitudes regarding asthma in their children: Impact of an educational intervention in an Indian population. Pediatric Pulmonology. 2020;**55**:607-615

[9] Sigurdardottir AO, Svavarsdottir EK, Rayens MK, et al. Therapeutic conversations intervention in pediatrics. Are they of benefit for families of children with asthma? Nursing Clinics of North America. 2013;**48**:287-304

[10] Isik E, Fredland NM, Freysteinson WM. School and community-based nurse-led asthma interventions for school-aged children and their parents: A systematic literature review. Journal of Pediatric Nursing. 2018;**44**:107-114

[11] Walter H, Sadeque-Iqbal F, Ulysse R, et al. Effectiveness of school-based family asthma educational programs in quality of life and asthma exacerbations in asthmatic children aged 5 to 18. JBI Database of Systematic Reviews and Implementation Reports. 2016;**14**:113-138

[12] Clark NM, Shah S, Dodge JA, et al. An evaluation of asthma interventions for preteen students. Journal of School Health. 2010;**80**:80-87

[13] McGhan SL, Wong E, Sharpe HM, et al. L'éducation sur l'asthme pour les enfants: Le programme Roaring Adventures of Puff (RAP) améliore la qualité de vie. Canadian Respiratory Journal. 2010;**17**:67-73

[14] Mosnaim GS, Li H, Damitz M, et al. Evaluation of the Fight Asthma Now (FAN) program to improve asthma knowledge in urban youth and teenagers. Annals of Allergy, Asthma, & Immunology. 2011;**107**:310-316

[15] Celano MP, Holsey CN, Kobrynski LJ. Home-based family intervention for low-income children with asthma: A randomized controlled pilot study. Journal of Family Psychology. 2012;**26**:171-178

[16] Payrovee Z, Kashaninia Z, Mahdaviani SA, et al. Effect of family

empowerment on the quality of life of school-aged children with asthma. Tanaffos. 2014;**13**:35-42

[17] Fouda LM, El-zeftawy AMA, Mohammed A, et al. Effect of family empowerment on the quality of life of school-aged children with asthma attending pediatric outpatient clinics of Tanta University and El-Mehalla El-Koubra Chest Hospital. International Journal of Advanced Research. 2015;**3**:346-360

[18] Grover C, Goel N, Armour C, et al. Medication education program for Indian children with asthma: A feasibility study. Nigerian Journal of Clinical Practice. 2015;**19**:76-84

[19] Arikan-Ayyildiz Z, Işık S, Çağlayan-Sözmen Ş, et al. Efficacy of asthma education program on asthma control in children with uncontrolled asthma. Turkish Journal of Pediatrics. 2016;**58**:383

[20] Canino G, Shrout PE, Vila D, et al. Effectiveness of a multi-level asthma intervention in increasing controller medication use: A randomized control trial. Journal of Asthma. 2016;**53**:301-310

[21] Yeh HY, Ma WF, Huang JL, et al. Evaluating the effectiveness of a family empowerment program on family function and pulmonary function of children with asthma: A randomized control trial. International Journal of Nursing Studies. 2016;**60**:133-144

[22] Kashaninia Z, Payrovee Z, Soltani R, et al. Effect of family empowerment on asthma control in school-age children. Tanaffos. 2018;**17**:47-52

[23] Mosenzadeh A, Ahmadipour S, Mardani M, et al. The effect of self-care education on the quality of life in children with allergic asthma. Comprehensive Child and Adolescent Nursing. Epub ahead of print 2 October 2018. DOI: 10.1080/24694193.2018.1513098

[24] Montalbano L, Ferrante G, Cilluffo G, et al. Targeting quality of life in asthmatic children: The MyTEP pilot randomized trial. Respiratory Medicine. 2019;**153**:14-19

[25] Dardouri M, Sahli J, Ajmi T, et al. Effect of family empowerment education on pulmonary function and quality of life of children with asthma and their parents in Tunisia: A randomized controlled trial. Journal of Pediatric Nursing. 2020;**54**:e9-e16

[26] Dardouri M, Bouguila J, Sahli J, et al. Assessing the impact of a family empowerment program on asthma control and medication use in children with asthma: A randomized controlled trial. Journal for Specialists in Pediatric Nursing. 2021;**e12324**:1-9

[27] Kocaaslan EN, Akgün KM. Effect of disease management education on the quality of life and self-efficacy levels of children with asthma. Journal for Specialists in Pediatric Nursing; **24**. [Epub ahead of print 1 April 2019]. DOI: 10.1111/jspn.12241

[28] Bindler R, Cowen K, Ball J. Clinical Skills Manual for Principles of Pediatric Nursing: Caring for Children. 5th ed. 2011. Available from: https://www.amazon.com/Clinical-Skills-Principles-Pediatric-Nursing/dp/0132625342. [Accessed: November 22, 2020]

[29] The National Heart Lung and Blood Institute. Expert Panel Report 3: Guidelines for the Diagnosis and Management of Asthma. Elsevier. Epub ahead of print 1 November 2012. DOI: 10.1016/j.jaci.2007.09.043

[30] Scottish Intercollegiate Guidelines Network and, British Thoracic Society. British Guideline on the Management of Asthma. 2019. Available from: www.brit-thoracic.org.uk

[31] The World Bank Group. World Bank Country and Lending Groups—Country Classification. 2020. Available from: https://datahelpdesk.worldbank.org/knowledgebase/articles/906519-world-bank-country-and-lending-groups. [Accessed: November 25, 2020]